"Katy Bowman has done it once again. Her books and articles are always cutting-edge sources of practical advice that is easy to implement, and *Whole Body Barefoot* is no exception! As a barefoot/minimalist shoe advocate myself, I often struggle with guiding my clients through the often confusing process of making the transition without injury. But now I have a done-for-you guide that shows exactly how it's done, from strengthening to stretching to shoe choice and more! This is a must-have book for anyone with feet."

—**Ben Greenfield**, athlete and author of the *New York Times* Best Seller *Beyond Training: Mastering Endurance, Health and Life*

"Her detailed approach to understanding barefoot biomechanics is impressive on its own, but there is much more. Katy does a wonderful job of offering useful exercises alongside constructive critique, and an absorbable lesson in physiology. This insightful book will lead you to clearly understand that it is not the product you do or do not use, but rather the role you play in your physical health. Read it."

—**Eric Goodman**, DC, Founder of Foundation Training

"Whether you're playing field sports or simply moving through daily life, success begins from the ground up. *Whole Body Barefoot* explains the 'why' and provides the 'how-to' in a logical, step-by-step plan to treat your feet and help you to move better."

—**Chip Morton**, Pro Football Strength & Conditioning Coach, Cincinnati, Ohio

T0161249

"As an endurance sports coach, most ailments I see can be linked to the feet. I am always looking for resources to provide athletes with practical reasons and solutions to common foot-related issues—such as 'duck feet' and over-pronation—and this book is one of the best I've found!

Once again, Katy inspires us to take charge of our body's 'shape' and be proactive instead of reactive—and exercise alone won't cut it. Whether you're a clinician or amateur athlete, *Whole Body Barefoot* is a comprehensive guide on biomechanics, anatomy and movement that will make us all more aware and stronger from the feet up! I even discovered new things about my feet and form in this book, and will be putting to use Katy's step-by-step guides on standing correctly, corrective exercises, and more."

—**Tawnee Prazak**, MS, CSCS, endurance sports coach, strength training specialist, athlete, and host of the *Endurance Planet* podcast

"*Whole Body Barefoot* delivers by taking the complex, whole-body, biomechanical issues of barefoot running and making it digestible for runners looking to begin barefoot running. I would highly recommend individuals looking to engage in barefoot running to read this book."

—**Joshua Stone**, MA, ATC, PES, CES

"In *Whole Body Barefoot*, Katy Bowman clearly outlines how most footwear changes the natural shape of our feet, and by extension, the function of our entire body. By applying the principles she teaches, you will be able to restore your foundation and prevent dysfunction. This the best form of healing, and it is for all of us."

—**Ray McClanahan**, DPM, creator of Correct Toes®

"Most people in the Paleo community have tried switching to more minimalist footwear, with varied success. Unfortunately, a lot of these new converts revert back to 'regular' shoes after experiencing increased foot pain, back problems and plantar fasciitis. If only these poor folks had this book! *Whole Body Barefoot* is an indispensable guide for anyone looking to make the successful transition to minimalist footwear, with the added bonus of improving the function of their entire body!"

— **Cain Credicott**, *Paleo Magazine*

"As Katy Bowman knowledgeably—and often humorously—explains, the concepts of barefoot biomechanics and minimal footwear aren't just about feet. *Whole Body Barefoot* offers a nuanced discussion of minimal shoes as just one potential component of a whole-body solution to what so often is really a whole-body problem."

— **Jordana Bieze Foster**, Editor, *Lower Extremity Review Magazine*

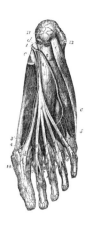

WHOLE
BODY
BAREFOOT

TRANSITIONING WELL TO
MINIMAL FOOTWEAR

KATY BOWMAN, M.S.

UPHILL
BOOKS

ALSO BY KATY BOWMAN

Rethink Your Position
Grow Wild
Dynamic Aging
Simple Steps to Foot Pain Relief
Movement Matters
Diastasis Recti
Don't Just Sit There
Move Your DNA
Alignment Matters

Printed in the United States of America.

Eighth Printing, 2023
ISBN-13: 9780989653985
Library of Congress Control Number: 2014957182

Uphill Books: uphill-books.com

Cover design: Melissa Jacobson
Interior design: Zsofi Koller, liltcreative.co
Illustrations: Jillian Nicol
Cover images: Mahina Hawley; J. Jurgensen Photography; iStock: Laurence Berger; Xero Shoes photo by Alexandra Kahn, PlanIt Vision Branding
Anatomical illustrations: Vector Hut, Creative Market and istockphoto/ ilbusca
Interior photography: J. Jurgensen Photography
Stone-walking image, pages 107 and 146: Ricardo Nagaoka
Shoe photo credits, pp xiv-xvi: Manitobah.ca (photo #1); Zaqq.com (2); EarthRunners.com (3); BeLenka.com (4); AtlantisHandmade.com (5); SoftstarShoes.com (6,9); LemsShoes.com (7,11); XeroShoes.com (8,12); OrigoShoes.com (10)

The information in this book should not be used for diagnosis or treatment, or as a substitute for professional medical care. Please consult with your health care provider prior to attempting any treatment on yourself or another individual.

Publisher's Cataloging-in-Publication
(Provided by Cassidy Cataloguing Services, Inc.).

Names: Bowman, Katy, author. | Nicol, Jillian Eve, 1982- illustrator.
Title: Whole body barefoot : transitioning well to minimal footwear / Katy Bowman, M.S. ; illustrations: Jillian Nicol.
Description: [Sequim, Washington] : Uphill Books, [2015] | Includes bibliographical references and index.
Identifiers: ISBN: 978-0-9896539-8-5 (paperback) | 978-0-9896539-2-3 (ebook) | LCCN: 2014957182
Subjects: LCSH: Footwear--Health aspects. | Shoes--Health aspects. | Foot--Movements. | Gait in humans. | Posture. | Exercise. | BISAC: HEALTH & FITNESS / Exercise / Stretching. | HEALTH & FITNESS / Exercise / General. | SPORTS & RECREATION / Walking. | SPORTS & RECREATION / Running & Jogging.
Classification: LCC: RA779 .B69 2015 | DDC: 613.482--dc23

For TP, whose footprints are everywhere I go.

CONTENTS

MINIMAL SHOES ARE FOR EVERY BODY, INCLUDING YOURS

You're about to dive into an entire book about minimal footwear. Maybe you came to this book as an athlete who depends on your feet for your sport, or maybe you're reading because your feet don't feel good most days and you have a hunch your footwear might be part of the problem. Either way, the reason for transitioning to minimal footwear is the same: improve the strength, performance, and longevity of the feet.

There are many stages to life, like childhood, middle age, and older adulthood. Injury and disease are also unavoidable stages of being human, and these can fall anywhere on our personal timeline. No matter your age or stage, having stronger feet will serve you better than having weak feet. That being said, certain features of a minimal shoe might work for you more than others depending on your personal movement history, your goals, and how you spend your day.

For example, one characteristic of a minimal shoe is that it doesn't stop your feet from feeling the shape of the ground. Thin, flexible soles let more movement in. But what if your work involves standing in place for many hours, or logging lots of steps on hard concrete? In these cases, blocking out some of the floor's hardness might be a wise choice. Does this mean you can't wear more minimal shoes to work? No. It means that you look for shoes that have some elements of "minimal footwear" while still providing you with the right amount of cushion or sole-thickness for your particular environment. You could also have certain shoes for your work environment and others with more flexible soles for time away from work.

I've been wearing minimal footwear for over fifteen years, but in 2023 when dealing with my own foot injury, I had to trade in my favorite thin and flexible running sandals for a thicker and stiffer-soled minimal athletic shoe for a few months while I was healing. When my body needed more support, I didn't need to ditch minimal footwear altogether; I just needed shoes that sat in a different place on the spectrum of minimal footwear.

I'm going to refer to minimal shoes a lot going forward, but keep this in mind: a "minimal shoe" is just a shoe that meets certain criteria—it's no one single shape, and each shoe is definitely not a "one-size-fits all." Below are some examples of footwear that are all "minimal" in that they're flat, have adequate space for toe movement, and fully attach to your foot (you'll learn more about that in the introduction). Not only is their sole thinness and flexibility on a spectrum, but you can also see the range in design.

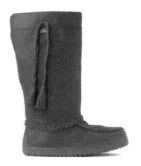

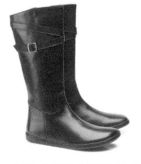

THICKER-SOLED WINTER BOOT   **THINNER-SOLED DRESS BOOT**

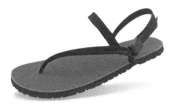

THICKER-SOLED SANDAL

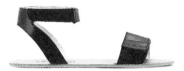

THINNER-SOLED SANDAL

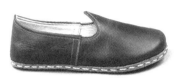

LOAFER

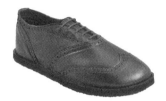

OXFORD

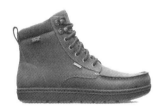

HIKING BOOT

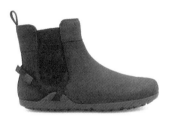

CHELSEA-STYLE BOOT

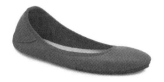

SIMPLE FLAT

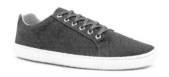

NO-HEEL SNEAKER

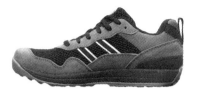 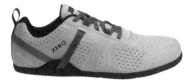

THICKER-SOLED ATHLETIC SHOE **THINNER-SOLED ATHLETIC SHOE**

This variety in minimal footwear shape means not only can we find the shoe that works best for our body, but also there are shoes for different seasons and situations too. There is minimal footwear that fits each area of your life.

If you start lifting weights to improve the strength of different body parts, you need to begin with the right load—not too little, and not too much. The same idea applies to selecting shoes. You will do well to keep in mind there is no single type of shoe that defines a "minimal shoe"; rather, "going minimal" is finding the minimal shoe characteristics that work best for you and where you are right now, and continuing to self-assess based on the progress you make on your physical journey. Just as you transition to minimal shoes in the first place, you will continue to transition between types of minimal shoes for the rest of your life depending on your current physical condition and environment. Putting on a more padded shoe because you're standing on hard floors every day isn't failing; it's being attuned to your needs and surroundings. So there's no "best minimal shoe." Instead, think: which shoe is right for you, right now?

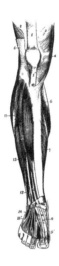

INTRODUCTION

I'm sure a lot of people probably anticipate that a minimal footwear book by the author of multiple books on natural movement and foot health would go something like "Minimal shoes are amazing. We should all be wearing them all the time and we'd all be healthier. The end."

Surprise! You will not find such a broad-stroke recommendation here. In fact, I'm writing this book because the opposite might be true: an incautious change to minimal footwear could very easily result in injury and further disease. I am, of course, a huge fan of minimal shoes, and I *do* think that everyone should be working towards eliminating conventional shoes from their closets. However, wearing minimal shoes without creating or prolonging injury and disease can require hundreds of steps (pun intended) along the way.

Our lives are crazy busy, and we like things to be laid out for us in simple steps. But this current culture of reducing necessary steps for health to five-foods-five-exercises-five-minutes-a-day lists means that important physiological guidelines get ignored in favor of being published in a magazine or on a website. I've been asked to create this kind of list many times—and yes, I've done it. Unfortunately, despite being initially helpful, a short list leaves out much of the work necessary to make meaningful health changes. In the case of the trendy move toward minimal shoes— where many hopped right in without doing any transitional work along the way—the result was an inevitable backlash when the shoes "didn't work like they were supposed to."

Minimal shoes, with their stated or implied ability to provide

---

WALK BEFORE YOU RUN

Thanks to *Born to Run* author Christopher McDougall and other barefoot-running proponents, many people hope to transition to minimal shoes for the purposes of running in a different way. If this is you, please remember that because the loads to your body (and feet) differ when you're running versus walking, they are entirely different things biomechanically speaking. While running is entirely natural (found in nature), natural running is performed by animals (including people) that have spent large amounts of time walking (and some health benefit to the wearer while performing an athletic endeavor, are surrounded by controversy. Without data on long-term users of footwear that is without support or cushioning, many medical practitioners have worried about injury. Minimal shoe companies and barefoot-running proponents have argued that being barefoot is natural and therefore barefoot shoes must be good. What has been clear to me, as someone who works to disseminate complex scientific information to laypeople without destroying its accuracy, is that much of this disagreement boils down to semantics and broad generalizations. And so, this book.

As with most arguments, when you examine this one closely, both sides are right *and* wrong. Research shows that minimal shoes are not safe for everyone in every situation—but research also shows that conventional shoes wreak their own havoc on the body.

The element that seems to be missing from the argument is that shoes don't exist in a vacuum. Shoes and feet are in a

---

squatting, and doing a ton of other non-running movements)—throughout a day, over a lifetime. Which means the strength and shapes of tissue you would naturally be bringing to a "barefoot" run would be affected by copious amounts of barefoot walking—walking that you haven't been doing. In the same way your toddler-body spent lots of time learning to walk before reflexively attempting running, you need to be building a running foundation that's larger than just running. For this reason, I'm going to talk about walking a lot more than running.

relationship with the user and the environment, which means the physical outcome of the body that wears the shoes depends on the state of the wearer's foot, body alignment, gait patterns, frequency of movement, and most-frequented terrain. A shoe can't be a problem *or* a solution in and of itself, and if we are going to determine what constitutes optimal footwear, we need to consider what's going on throughout the user's body and life.

Both sides of the minimal shoe debate want what they believe is best—most healthy—for the population. (Let's just ignore the debaters with serious intere$t in the minimal footwear game and those who just like to snicker about the appearance of minimal shoes. I have no idea whether or not these groups have your best outcomes in mind.) Still, both sides could use a broader perspective and a longer discussion than typically happens on social media. To clarify language is to clarify an argument.

So, before I get into the details regarding *how* to transition, I want to clarify—in detail—just what we are transitioning to.

The term *minimal footwear* (also referred to as minimalist footwear, or barefoot shoes) as I use it means a shoe that minimizes its alteration of natural human movement. This is a slightly different interpretation from the term *minimal* as applied to the quantity of materials making up the shoe. For example, a flip-flop is perceived, by many, to be a minimal shoe because of its low shoe-mass. But with in-depth biomechanical analysis, or even superficial biomechanical analysis (i.e., just look down at your feet when you're walking in flip-flops), you can see that a flip-flop alters the way you walk (as explained in Chapter One). Which means that simply having minimal mass isn't the best characteristic by which to classify a shoe as "minimal."

Shoes are typically broken down into four components known to impact human performance (that is, to perform the biological functions necessary to be human, not to win a race): sole, heel, upper, and toe-box.

Minimal shoes have:

- a sole that is thin and flexible enough for the tissues in the foot (and not just the ankle) to feel the ground below the foot and respond by articulating, innervating, contracting, releasing, etc.;

- a heel that is neutral, or "zero-drop," allowing all joints to work from a neutral baseline and enabling the full range of motion for all joints in the body;

- an upper that fully connects the foot to the shoe, so there's no need to grip the toes or the front of the shin to keep the shoe on while walking;

- a spacious toe-box that allows enough room for the toes to extend and spread as necessary while walking, hiking, or climbing; and

- a front of the shoe that rests on the ground (as opposed to one that swoops upward and raises the front of the shoe above the standing surface, slightly extending the toes).

Minimal footwear is not about being as tiny as possible; minimal footwear allows your feet to behave as feet while still offering a buffer between the unnatural detritus found in the modern world that can cause injury.

Shoes are shaping the humans who wear them—and not for the better. This is why I am most interested in footwear. I deal with the injured public, individuals with head-to-toe ailments that they've been trying to remedy for years (and for thousands of dollars) with little or no success. Thwarted by what they put on their feet each morning and stomp around in all day, well-intentioned folks go to the chiropractor's office, spinal surgeon, and podiatrist looking for answers to the wrong question. The question is not "How can I fix this?" but "What am I doing every day to create this?"

Your shoes and how you use them can limit the full "nutritional spectrum" created through movement. You have thirty-three joints in each foot, and the muscle groups of the feet make up twenty-five percent of the body's total number of muscles. The complex machinery of the feet plays a critical role not only in the obvious realms of gait patterns and ankle stabilization but also in whole-body balance, nerve conduction, and cardiovascular circulation. Your shoes are affecting a whole lot more than your outfit—they're capping the limits of your health. That professional footwear you're selecting each day is the glass ceiling to your well-being.

I've already written an entire book on the human foot, foot pain, and the effects of shoes (*Simple Steps for Foot Pain Relief: The New Science of Healthy Feet*). After people read it, the most common question about the footwear guidelines and the shoe recommendations is always something along the lines of "I get what you're saying about shoes and the feet and alignment in general, but I have specific foot condition X, so what do I need to do, specifically?" Our prescription-oriented medical culture makes us think that we all need a different medicine for our ailments—that what works for most feet will certainly not work for our own because of our special issues. What we don't understand is that nearly all of these myriad problems are stemming from a cultural problem: there's a baseline of movement that we are *all* missing, and our bodies are responding in different ways to the same lack of movement. Once we restore that movement in our lives, our body restores its own equilibrium or homeostasis, eliminating the problems that can seem so unique.

Say your daily water consumption is one cup of water per day.

Eventually your lack of water leads to constipation, and so you buy my book titled *Healing Yourself with Water* (this is a fake book title—I am not an expert on drinking water) and skim the entire thing, looking for the place where I talk about constipation, specifically, and how much water *you* need to drink to fix *your* problem.

But let's say I spend the first half of the book explaining how water works and how the human body requires eleven cups a day to stay hydrated and function properly. By doing this I've effectively told every single person exactly what they need to get better. To make it apply to you, all you have to do is subtract the number of cups of water you were drinking before (one, in this case) from eleven, and BAM, you have your personal recommendation (drink ten more cups of water a day). Do I really have to write, "If you drink two cups a day, then add nine more" and "If you drink seven cups a day, then add four more"? Do I have to say, "If you are constipated, you need eleven cups of water a day; if you are not constipated, you need eleven cups of water a day"?

Also, the experience we have regarding our health couldn't possibly be the result of any one thing. Rather, each of us is a physical ball of habits, environments, and scenarios. The water you drink is just one input. (Which means that constipation isn't caused by drinking only one cup of water. Some people get constipated even when they drink six or eight cups of water!) There's no possible way to write a book that meets every individual right where they are without giving a framework based on the biological essentials. Maybe your water is disease-ridden—and then it's not the quantity you need to adjust, but the quality. Again, my fake book covers the essentials of water drinking, but it doesn't address every single variable in every single reader's life.

I can probably stop extending this metaphor—you get it, right? Don't thumb through this book just for a section on plantar fasciitis or bunions. The whole book applies to you— every book I've written applies to you—because you have a body, and my work deals in the essential movements required for human bodies to be healthy and to thrive. You want to know which habits need modification, which exercises you need to do, and what you need to learn with respect to what goes on your feet? You need to read, learn, and do all of this stuff. The end.

But not quite the end, sorry. Before I close out this intro- duction, which is really just the beginning, I need to say this: There are many wonderful things about shoes. Humans have been wearing foot coverings, probably for eons, to great results. Protection from cold has allowed us to migrate beyond the confines of year-round comfortable weather. Protective soles have given our minds a certain freedom from the constant monitoring necessary to avoid wounds. But whenever we use technology—yes, shoes are technology—we pay a biological tax. For wearing shoes, we pay that tax not just with our feet but with our entire bodies. Transitioning to minimal footwear isn't necessary only to decrease foot disease. Our bodies cannot function optimally unless our feet are in good shape, which means we need to stop outsourcing the body's work to inani- mate objects. The move to minimal shoes is a move towards a stronger body, which in turn is a huge step (stop it with the puns already!) toward whole-body health.

CULTURAL SHOES

Many of the features found in modern shoes, like heels or a narrow toe-box, are there for cultural reasons—they change with fashion. The idea of what we need in a shoe, and why we need shoes, is also tainted with a cultural perspective based on ideas about the superiority of certain cultures and classes. In many cases, someone who wasn't wearing shoes was considered savage and/or lesser—whether it was a street urchin in London or an indigenous person in the "New World." A lack of shoes was equated with savagery—a sort of primitive behavior (setting aside the obvious fact that we are, of course, primates).

In many cultures, wearing shoes was once a way to signify the distance between the shoe-wearer and shoe-free cultures and classes in the same way that pale skin was valued for its "indooredness" (darkened skin was an indication of outside work), using a wet nurse or infant formula were promoted over a mother breastfeeding, and chairs were used in lieu of dirt-floor sitting. Shoes (and furniture, bottles, toilets, etc.) were often a sign not just of civilization, but of being more civilized than another group.

THINK MORE ABOUT YOUR FEET

- Did you ever go barefoot when you were a kid? What are your memories of that?

- What's your earliest memory about shoes?

- When was the last time you remember feeling comfortable walking barefoot?

- How do your feet feel every day?

- Do any of your shoes hurt your feet?

- Do any of your shoes feel great?

- Does your workplace or social setting dictate which shoes you wear?

- Does the sensation in your feet ever stop you from doing what you want to do?

- What makes your feet feel fantastic?

- Where would you like to go barefoot right now?

- What's something you'd like to do when your feet are stronger?

THINK

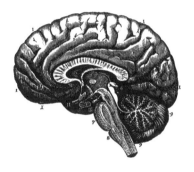

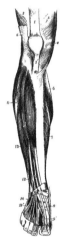

CHAPTER ONE

FOOTWEAR

Imagine you ate a diet crafted entirely out of foods available at a movie theater. Popcorn, soda, candy, and maybe a plate of fake-cheese nachos every now and then. On one hand, in terms of "getting as many calories as you need," the movie theater diet poses no problem at all. You have food! Amazing. But unless some of that junk food was vitamin C–enhanced, you'd soon find yourself with scurvy. You'd eventually run low on B12; you'd be weak and tired and your digestion would begin to fall apart. You'd become iron-deficient, perhaps developing a swollen and sore tongue or brittle fingernails. Your diet would not include what we now recognize as good (essential) fats. Your pancreas probably couldn't keep up with your sugar intake. Really, I could craft a list of ailments to go with each missing nutrient as well as a list of ailments that correlate with the excessive consumption of whatever is found in these foods. The list of problems with an all-junk-food diet is equal in length to the nutrients essential to our well-being. Our health is made of the inputs that we both do and don't get.

If you asked me, "What's the problem with an all junk-food diet?" the answer could go on forever. But in a nutshell I could say that the input isn't what your body requires, and that without the correct input, your body will fail over time. On the other hand, given the right context—there is no other food around, for example—you could argue logically (using scientific evidence!) that the movie-theater diet is life-saving.

Similarly, conventional footwear can't be reduced to one single problem, as each aspect of a shoe does something different to the body. Each shoe feature potentially changes the input created by moving. In some cases, the reduction of input—like a nail or a piece of glass—is welcome. In other cases, the reduction of input—like to the sensory nerves in the feet, for example—isn't so good, especially when this reduction has been experienced over a lifetime. Tissues atrophy and die in the absence of input.

In general, conventional footwear is narrower than the foot in its unshod state, has an elevated heel, and is stiff- and thick-soled. Shoes can press the toes together, which weakens foot musculature, thereby affecting nerve health. Elevated heels make it impossible to access the full range of motion of many joints—which in turn creates highly repetitive but small motions in the hips and knees. And because all of your parts are connected, you have to make constant adjustments to the pelvis and spine in order to stay upright while you're essentially walking downhill (your toes are below your ankles, thanks to your heeled shoes) on flat ground. Don't get me wrong, adjusting your body to go downhill is no problem—it's one of the reasons you come with so many hinges. But consider that you've been walking on some degree of decline almost every step of your life, which has forced your body to adjust not only its position but its mass distribution and pressure system—all to cope with this "heel" input. See what I mean? Shoes impact the body in many different ways.

The good news is that the very fact that there are so many different problems with shoes actually makes "getting healthier" a bit easier; you can slowly change portions of your body *and* your shoes over time, which keeps the transition from becoming overwhelming.

When it comes to transitioning out of traditional footwear, everyone needs to begin with a shoe variable that makes sense to their own body. As far as whole-body impact goes, I have found working to eliminate the heel the most important step. However, if you've got achy, grippy toes, you might want to consider ditching your clogs, mules, or flip-flops, and finding a shoe that has a more attached upper. Or maybe you've never worn positive-heeled shoes but still have weak feet, or ankles that pronate, and you feel like you need heavy-duty arch support in order for your feet to be comfortable. In that case you'll benefit greatly from the strengthening and habitual positioning exercises and guidelines in the Move section—and you'll probably need to change up the kinds of surfaces you walk on.

I've been teaching people about shoes, feet, and gait for over a decade, and I've found that understanding the basic geometry of footwear helps people understand the mechanical changes to the body that shoes and walking in shoes over a lifetime can bring about, and why and how the body adapts to different shoe input.

THE HEEL

What is a heel?

A heel as I'm using the term is any elevation in the back half of a shoe. Many people claim they don't wear heels, but unless you've already been purposefully seeking out completely flat footwear, chances are you've been wearing heels. Walk into any shoe store and look at any style of shoe, from "flats" to athletic shoes to sturdy winter boots, never mind the *actual* "heels," and chances are you'll find an elevated heel.

Truly, a heel in and of itself is no problem. The body, as I mentioned before, comes with all the equipment necessary (hinges and levers) to adjust to changing gradients underneath the feet. But what about when *all* of your shoes have been heeled for *all* of your life?

HEELS AND "BODY NEUTRAL"

" Wearing barefoot shoes was a critical part of my recovery from fourteen years of chronic pelvic pain. After learning how to walk differently with [your exercises], I would walk for hours in barefoot shoes through Weston-super-Mare woods and along the beach. I could feel my glutes and pelvic floor working with each step. Walking over rough terrain also allowed my feet to become supple. It seems strange that after paying for so many different, expensive treatments for pelvic pain, doing something so simple could make such a huge difference to my body."

DAVID MCCOID

Many proponents of minimal footwear—specifically those calling for heel elimination—use a graphic similar to this one.

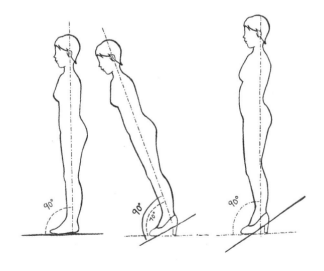

While a version of this image is used a lot, I don't think the information conveyed by the image is clear to everyone—and it needs to be, if you're trying to quantify just how much your whole body is impacted by a heel. So, lemmebreakitdownforya.

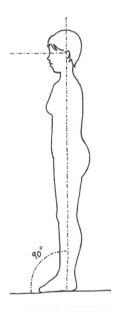

PICTURE A

In Picture A (above) we have a barefoot person whose neutral body position lines up perpendicularly to the ground. This is helpful when it comes to figuring out loads—that is, how parts are squished between the head and the feet.

Now that the figure is wearing shoes, the "ground" (if we define *ground* as whatever the body is standing on) has changed, which means that the body-neutral axis is now perpendicular relative to the new ground (picture B, below).

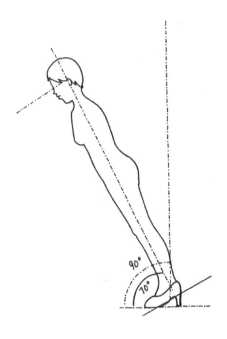

PICTURE B

Of course, the body can't stand in this way, and THANK GOODNESS you have joints that can articulate to keep you upright when you're going downhill. However, the body responds—continuously—to mechanical input. And what biomechanists, physical therapists, orthopedists, and YOU should be concerned with is the load created by this new surface. How does your body have to compensate for this new ground you are walking upon? What new input is created when you right yourself so that you can, in fact, walk around?

This is where Picture C comes in:

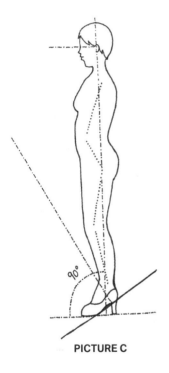

PICTURE C

In order to bring your body—your head, actually—upright, you have to move your body backward relative to your standing surface (which is the plane established by points under the ball of your foot and your heel). This picture communicates a scenario in which the shin stays forward, more in line with the shoe-ground, with the backward motion coming at the knee and ribcage—creating a particular angle in the legs and spine. This is one way of coping with shoes; the resulting shape of the body can be any combination of backward motion of the joints between the ankles and head.

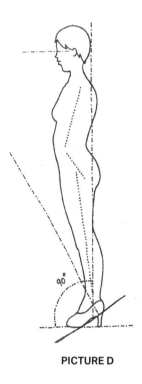

PICTURE D

Picture D (above) illustrates a different way one can "straighten up" while wearing heels. It's challenging for researchers to pinpoint exactly what happens when you wear a heel, because what happens depends on the shape and mass distributions of your particular body plus your preferred way to

compensate. This is one of the reasons research on shoe characteristics can conflict; people are all shaped and behave uniquely,
even within particular demographics.

And menfolk, just because this graphic ALWAYS features
women, doesn't mean that the same thing isn't going on in your
body when you wear heeled shoes. The only difference is that the
heels on men's shoes tend not to be as high as the ones in this
graphic and their feet tend to be longer (see Picture E, below). On
the other hand, men tend to be four inches taller (on average)

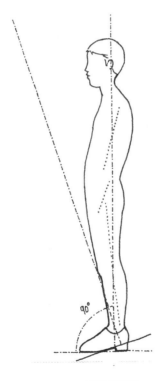

PICTURE E

KIDS AND HEELED SHOES

Recalling Picture B on page 20, there are three measures that affect how much a heel distorts a body from neutral: the height of the heel, the length of the foot, and the height of the body.

The shorter the foot wearing a heeled shoe, the greater the angle upon which the foot is set. When it comes to putting kids in heeled shoes, it bears emphasizing:

- The higher the heel, the more forward the body is projected.

- The shorter the foot, the more forward the body is projected.

- The taller the body, the more forward the body is projected.

Kids are short, but they also have short feet, which is why it drives me crazy to see a child's shoe with a heel the same height as their parents'. The short foot of a child "magnifies" a heel's effect—even a heel of seemingly inconsequential height. Which means that, in the case of the shoes pictured (a woman's size 7 and a child's size 8.5), the angle between

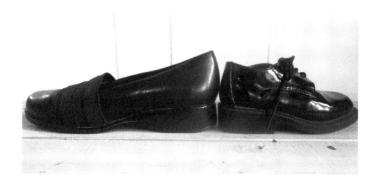

than women, which means your long body will be distorted more than a woman of lesser height wearing the same shoe size.

Here's why this is important: Even though it seems like you're standing upright on top of shoes, the loads to your body are very different than they would be if you were standing unshod on level ground.

When you consider, as I do, the body as a collection of cells that are individually responding to mechanical input, and how a cell's response to its mechanical environment results in a particular genetic expression (read my book *Move Your DNA* for the big-picture topics of mechanotransduction and diseases of captivity), then heels become very important to the discussion.

No matter how you stack up personally, consider how each

---

the standing surface and the foot would be much greater in the child than in the adult. It also means that the necessary compensation to get the body back "upright" is relatively greater for the child than the adult. Want to experience the math for yourself? Go to a free-standing bookshelf and put this book under either the right or left side to see how far the bookshelf tips. (For extra fun, look how the books shift and imagine how the loads to each of the "book cells" change in this arrangement.) Then put this book under the back of the bookshelf and again, note the total distance traveled by the unit...and the books. Barring medical conditions or the occasional dress up, heeled shoes have no place in a child's wardrobe. Children's shoes are not mini versions of adult fashion; they're maxi versions. They *amplify* the deleterious effects of traditional footwear. For this reason (and for many others), we seek out minimal shoes for our kids.

---

cell's mechanical environment compares in pic A and C. Yes, a change in position requires bones to move, but it also requires muscles to shorten and lengthen. And some parts are not pressed against each other (or the ground) as much as they could have been. Cells within bones become compressed (or not), resulting in a particular bone-mass distribution. While the effects of loads are subtle, these subtle deformations are what your cells (and then, your entire body) are adapting to.

Again, stacking yourself going downhill is totally natural; what's unnatural is the duration (all day, whole life) we've spent in the mechanical environment that is a heeled shoe. It's not just that your cells are, in a shoe with a heel, behaving differently than they would in a natural scenario. It's that they've behaved unnaturally almost every second of your waking and moving life.

THERE ARE MORE "PARTS" TO YOUR BODY THAN YOU REALIZE

The problem isn't only with the cellular squish. There are less subtle things going on when you have a heeled shoe, things you can see and measure with your very own eyes—like how you walk when you're wearing them.

In the same way a shoe "casts" the loads to your cells, the heel of a shoe prevents—quite clearly—your heel from reaching the ground. So what? This constant positioning of the heel above the forefoot changes the distances over which our individual parts work. Not the whole body, of course. The whole body still moves over the ground per usual, but how that motion gets done is

ONE MAN'S TRASH

Shoes bring many people relief from discomfort, and for that reason they have value. For example, one of the reasons people opt for heeled shoes is the slack a shoe's heel puts in the posterior muscle line that runs from the pelvis to the heel of the foot. Because we've been sitting the bulk of our lives *and* worn positive-heeled shoes since just about birth, the calf muscle running from the thigh to the Achilles tendon has adapted by shortening. When you put on a heeled shoe, it gives you a little slack in the posterior-leg muscles, taking some of the pressure off your lower back when you stand up.

While the heel can bring about relief for many, the problem—the slow loss of necessary tissue mass throughout the entire body—continues. Like all "orthotics" (and I'm using *orthotic* as a general term to mean something that supports some systems while preventing others from working), this temporary relief ends up turning off the alarm (back, knee, or heel pain) without correcting the problem. Takeaway: Use your orthotics—whatever they may be—as necessary, but don't mistake shutting off the alarm for putting out the fire.

changed when there is a structure blocking the ankle from participating fully, the way it would if there were no shoe.

When you're trying to troubleshoot/fix/build a machine, it helps to have a list of components or parts. If I had you name all the parts of the ankle, you could pull out your anatomy book and come up with a list that included tissue-structures like bone, muscle, tendon, and fascia. But if you're interested in having optimally functioning feet, and restoring the motions that are necessary for muscle development, circulation, and nerve health, your list of components must include the range of motion of the ankle as a "part" of the machine. And just like you'd list all the muscles and bones necessary for facilitating full movement, so then must you list every individual degree of the ankle's range of motion as its own part.

It might be challenging to consider "5 degrees of range of motion" to be a real part, but keep in mind that as mobility is lost, so is the ultimate function of the machinery of the foot—of any machine, really. Would you accept wheels on your car that only rotated 355°? When you consider every degree of range of motion as "necessary," then you can quickly see why heels don't work for long-term function. A heel effectively casts a portion of your potential range of motion, keeping this portion from participating when you stand or walk.

Furthermore, each of the muscles we put on our imaginary list of parts isn't really a single part at all. Each muscle-part is a structure made up of many tiny parts—parts that can be gained or lost through use. And when you lose one joint-range-of-motion part, you also lose one part of your muscle length. Walking with an elevated heel results, over time, in a loss of more parts than you were probably aware of: degrees of motion and lengths of muscle tissue.

This loss of tissue comes with a gain, but it's not a gain that lends itself to optimal long-term function of the legs. When the heel is prevented access to the ground, all other joints participate more. Again, this isn't necessarily a bad thing—joints are

OTHER WAYS CONVENTIONAL SHOES CAN SUCK (BIOMECHANICALLY SPEAKING)

- They have a too-tight toe-box that prevents toes from spreading and even crunches the toes together (think a pointy dress shoe).

- The upper doesn't connect with the foot (clogs, flip-flops).

- The sole is stiff and unyielding, forcing the work of walking to come from the ankle rather than being distributed throughout the foot, and also thick, so that the foot isn't distorted (read: moved at many of its thirty-three joints) by walking over shapes provided by the ground.

there to compensate for each other. But this particular compensation, in a natural environment, would be limited to a rise or drop in terrain that would quickly change. Our bodies' compensations as a whole are not long-term friendly, but are best used as short-term occurrences that are constantly changing with the terrain, in the case of the foot and ankle. Only, we don't walk on anything but flat ground for most of our steps. And the angle of our shoes is constant. Which means that our body equipment, which performs best in constantly changing conditions, has been allowed small ranges of motion at a very high frequency. And because every step you've ever taken has been using less of the ankle and more than what's natural of other joints, the muscles and ranges of motion that would have been used (and strengthened) by natural walking have not been, and joints that should not have been used for every step have—and they pay the price.

The effects of this loss/gain relationship don't just apply to the foot and ankle; the effects are whole-body. Once you start compensating, other joints become limited by proxy, other muscles' lengths are lost, and so on. And it's not all loss and shortening; the opposite is true for the opposing areas—imagine the front of the shin of a habitual heel-wearer. When a joint angle is held open for a longer duration than is natural, tissues have to change to accommodate this load. In many cases this brings about unnatural increases in joint laxity (commonly referred to as hypermobility) and in muscle length, which also limit ranges of strong and stabilized motion in a slightly different way.

Are there good heels and bad heels? No. There are just heels, no judgment. But every positive heel—even those that have been deemed "sensible"—impedes your body's full range of motion and affects the literal shape of your body. Which means that even if you work hard to live a movement-filled life of walking, squatting, and hanging (all the essential movements I recommend in *Move Your DNA*), if you do so wearing conventional running shoes with a half- to one-inch heel, you're not bringing all of your parts to the party.

TRANSITIONING OUT OF A HEEL

" Throwing out my heels was hard at first, until I started seeing the results. I had been suffering with low back and pelvis pain that kept me basically disabled for three years. After lots of PT and chiropractic work, my neurologist had told me I would fight some chronic back pain the rest of my life because at twenty-seven, I had a sixty-year-old back. I didn't think I wore a lot of heeled or problematic shoes, until I learned from Katy how I was perpetuating my own pain in my footwear choice. The results were so compelling and (relatively) quick that I was a hundred percent converted within a year, giving away every sentimental pair of "cute" shoes. In the three years since then I've seen my bunions heal by fifty percent on the bad foot, and almost completely on the other.

MARCEE MONROE LUDLOW

So you want to invite some of your old parts back to the party. Does that mean you should throw out your heels straight away? Nope. When you've worn a positive-heeled shoe the bulk of your life, your tiny parts are distributed differently than you need them to be in order to walk with your heels down. To transition abruptly is to run the risk of creating an injury. My first recommendation for moving away from a heel is to spend at least a month doing the correctives (exercises and habit modifications, found in the Move section) daily while continuing to wear your regular shoes. Yes, *even if* you regularly wear high heels.

ESPECIALLY if you wear heels every day, all day long. Focus on gradual changes in your shoes. Start working your (heel's) way down, but do it in stages. There are a number of "transitional" minimal shoes on the market now that offer an 8 millimeter or 4 millimeter heel rise. Slowly lowering the height of your shoes' heels while at the same time following the exercises laid out in this book is your best bet.

You'll know you're ready to progress to a lower heel height when you are able to go deeper with the calf stretch series, when it's easy for you to keep your pelvis from jutting forward, and when you can walk in lower-heeled shoes without pain.

THE FLIP-FLOP FLAW

Maybe you're a flip-flop lover feeling pretty relieved because your flip-flops seem minimal—flat, wide, and flexible. They're also "open"—an important component of the "natural" argument, as they allow for greater sensory input in the form of air pressure and temperature. It's true, flip-flops are SO CLOSE! But flip-flops fall short of being minimal-for-the-purpose-of-natural-gait in a vital way—they don't connect to our feet. We have to work our muscles unnaturally to keep them on. (Unfortunately, this toe-gripping action is necessary for slides, mules, and many slippers, too.) After a while, the toe-gripping motor pattern leads to shortened toe muscles (and a loss of parts that allow movement) which can then affect things like balance and foot arch strength, and lead to toe contractures, a.k.a.

hammertoes. New flip-flop research also shows that working to keep the shoe on changes many things about your gait, which means they end up affecting more than the feet.

I know, I know. Gripping doesn't sound like such a big deal, but gripping—when you're walking—is more than just toes bending in different places. Those bends end up changing which parts of the foot push into the ground. Those bends end up translating into mechanical input at the level of the nerves and skin and can create many problems not filed under "musculoskeletal."

Let me show you.

When you wear shoes that don't hold themselves on your foot, this is how the grip translates into buckling parts and pressures:

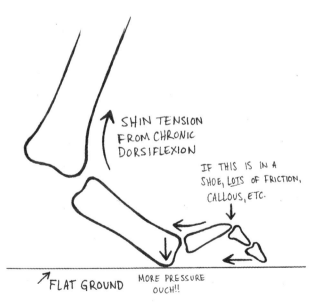

SHIN TENSION FROM CHRONIC DORSIFLEXION

IF THIS IS IN A SHOE, LOTS OF FRICTION, CALLOUS, ETC.

FLAT GROUND

MORE PRESSURE OUCH!!

The "grip" to keep footwear on curls some toe bones up and some down, drives the end of some bones into the ground, creating higher-than-normal pressure (which is what can lead to toe contracture/metatarsal injury over time), and drives the ends of some bones up into the top of the shoe (which can lead to corns and calluses over time if there's something for the toes to rub on overtop). I won't even mention the tension down the front of the leg—because you'll find it yourself during the Top of the Foot stretch in Chapter Five. (If you want to try that right now, go ahead. I'll wait.)

To keep your natural stride (and shoe) on *and* enjoy the feel of the sea breeze and sunshine on your skin, or the grit of dirt and the freezing cold air of a Canadian fall, opt for something that looks more like a Greek sandal. You know, all strappy and minimal but still fully connected to your foot. If you look around, you can find uppers that are very minimal as far as mass goes, but engineered in a way that keeps the shoe on without you needing to tighten your toes.

IT'S NOT *ONLY* THE SHOES

It's important to note that the tension in the calf—tension that results in heel pain for many—doesn't only stem from how your shoes fix your ankle into a slight toe point, but also from how a chair "casts" your knee at 90°. Which means that if a minimal-shoe-friendly body is what you're after, you should also reduce the amount of time you spend with your knees bent—a position that also shortens the posterior leg muscles. You'll find more on this as well as exercises to help in the Move section.

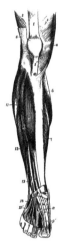

CHAPTER TWO

THE ANKLE

I've talked about some of the instant distortions that shoes can bring about. There is also longer-term physical distortion brought about by muscle strengths and weaknesses, in turn brought about by the distances you have walked (or haven't), how frequently you have sat (and how), and your shoe history over a lifetime.

You and I are part of a fully shod, sitting-most-of-the-time culture, and the effects go beyond tight hamstrings and calves, or bunions and hammertoes. Just like the flopped-over fin of an orca in captivity, our legs as a whole are collapsing at the hip—and taking the ankle with them. I've said it before and I'll say it again: foot health is a whole-body issue, and perhaps nothing demonstrates this as clearly as ankle schmear.

Ankle schmear is a term I coined myself, because I find it helps clarify what's actually going on structurally during a motion called pronation. You've probably heard of pronation—the "inward" roll of the foot while you're walking or running. Many an athletic shoe and orthotic has been devised to prevent this from happening and it's usually drawn like this:

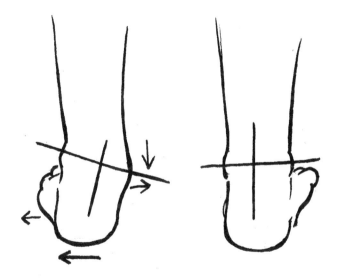

But pronation isn't really a tipping-inward motion—or more accurately, it isn't only a tipping-inward motion. Pronation is actually a tri-planar motion of the ankle complex, meaning that the bones in the lower leg and foot move and change orientation in three different planes, meaning we need to talk about planes now.

PLANE 1: Say you're going to spread some peanut butter onto a piece of bread and you start with the peanut butter on one side of the slice and move it to the other side.

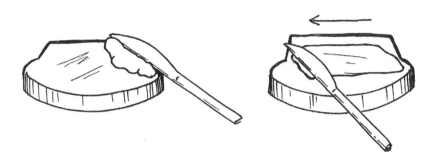

PLANE 2: When you spread the peanut butter from right to left, you're not only moving it across the bread, you're decreasing the height of the original pile as well.

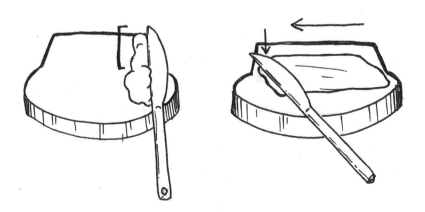

PLANE 3: Okay, so now pretend the knife's handle has been anchored at one end with a nail. In this case you would not able to spread stuff from right to left, but would be forced to spread the peanut butter from one side of the bread to the back edge of the bread by swinging the knife around the axis created by the nail:

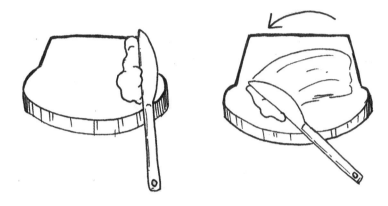

Voila! If you put those three motions together, you get pronation: a motion that rotates the shin inward (think knees pointing more towards each other), moves the leg toward the midline of the body, and lowers the leg a bit closer to the floor.

So now let's talk about schmear. While I do like to make up words (thank goodness for book editors), I didn't create the term *ankle schmear* just because I didn't like the term *pronation*. Schmear and pronation are different, and here's how: Pronation is the tri-planar movement I've described above and schmear is the *effect* of this triplanar distortion on the lower leg as a whole. You see, the foot and all its motions do not exist in a vacuum.

(P.S. If you're currently living in an actual vacuum that last sentence doesn't pertain to you.) The sole of your foot is in a physical relationship with the ground below it.

Because your foot skin is in traction between the ground below and the body above, when the leg rotates inward, the shin brings the top of the foot with it, pulling the top of the foot away from the bottom, which creates "extra mass" on the outer edge of the foot. With schmear, what you get is all parts of the foot distorted, both relative to the ground and to each other (see image below).

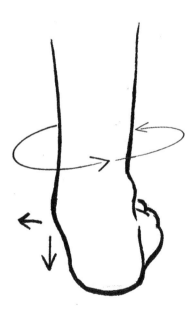

Understanding schmear will come in handy when you start lining up your feet only to find that you've got a bulk of mass extending beyond the outer edges of the foot. Yes, in many cases, when you look down at the top of your foot, you're staring at a portion of the bottom. Wait. What did you say? What just happened? Go back and read it again.

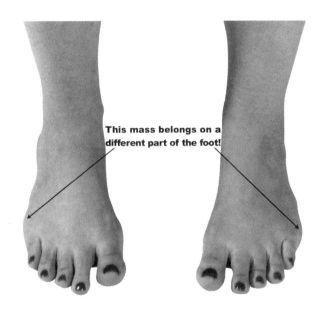

This mass belongs on a different part of the foot!

Isn't biomechanics fun?

So now you know that the bones of your feet can move within the foot-skin casing (thank goodness for the fascial system!), which may have you asking, "So what muscle can move my sole back under my foot?" And the answer is…there is no muscle in the foot that can get your foot-parts back to where they should be.

THE ANKLE JOINT COMPLEX

Most people think of the ankle joint as an up-and-down hinge, moving at those two quarter-sized bumps (called *malleoli*) just above your foot, but if we go a bit deeper we find movement in the "ankle" area to be more complex, hence the term *ankle joint complex*.

What we normally think of as the ankle is actually two joints: the talocrural (superiorly—closer to the head) and the subtalar (inferiorly—closer to the feet). Just looking at the two names, you see that both joints share the talus bone (Latin, for ankle). The "true" ankle, or talocrural joint, is made up of articulations between the tibia, fibula, and talus. The subtalar joint (aka the talocalcaneal joint) is made up of an anterior, middle, and posterior facet, and is what allows for the triplanar motion.

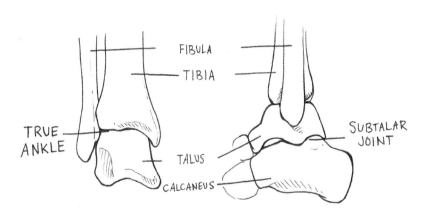

The "true" ankle joint brings about (dorsiflexion and plan-tarflexion) motion at the malleoli, but the subtalar joint below acts more like a gyroscope, allowing the body to walk upright even when walking over varied terrain.

Because our walking is primarily flat-and-level-ground walking, the dynamic function of the subtalar joint is less than what it would have been were we walking on varied terrain, and following suit, exploration into the universal

INFERIOR SURFACE OF TALUS

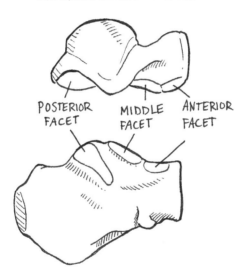

POSTERIOR FACET   MIDDLE FACET   ANTERIOR FACET

SUPERIOR SURFACE OF CALCANEUS

function of the ankle joint complex is less than what it should be. Meaning, research into the ankle complex has been skewed towards research into the "function of the ankle" as it functions on flat and level ground.

Rather, the foot skin has to be unschmeared by the reverse motion of the hip (external instead of internal rotation) while the foot skin is on the ground. Sole + traction + external rotation can change the foot skin, the loads to the foot bones, and the axis of the ankle joints in one fell swoop. Which is why I include this and other exercises to strengthen the hip rotators and lateral hip muscles in the Move section.

When you start working on changing your thigh position, as you'll find in the thigh-rotation exercise, there is an immediate change to the position of the hip, knee, ankle, and—because you're unschmearing—the height of the arch of the foot. And with foot-arch height can come a reduction in foot length.

LET'S CHECK IF YOUR SCHMEAR IS AFFECTING YOUR SHOE SIZE

“ After wearing minimalist shoes for four weeks and working intensely with [your exercises] I showed up to perform a concert. I did my usual switch from flat shoes into short heels shortly before the concert and realized within seconds that my feet hurt, that I couldn't balance my upper half over my lower half, and that there was a noticeable difference in my flute sound. So, I took the heels off, performed in the flats, and will never wear the heels again for a performance!

KELLY MOLLNOW WILSON

1. Stand on a piece of paper with your foot pointing straight forward, completely loaded. Keep your muscles relaxed. No need to correct anything yet (we want to see where your foot is most of the time).

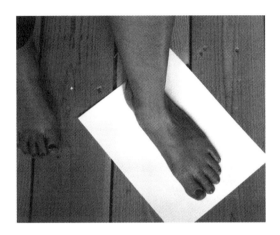

2. Trace around your foot.

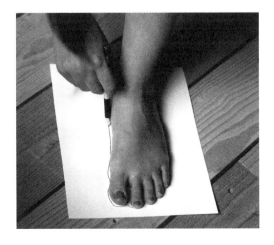

3. Step off and measure your foot length.

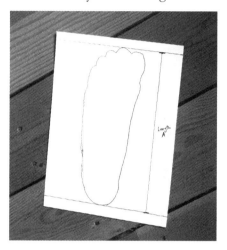

4. Place your foot back into your print and then externally rotate your thigh until your knee pit is in neutral (as described and pictured in Neutral Femurs on pages 64–65).

5. Retrace your foot.

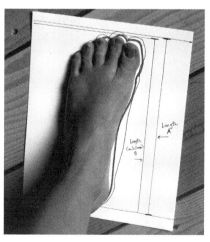

6. Highlight your "rotated thigh" foot with a different color and re-measure your length (or width or just shape in general). Here you can see that not only is my left foot (which always runs about quarter-inch longer than my right) shorter when my thigh and shin are less rotated off their axis, it is also narrower once I've undone the tri-planar distortion of my ankle complex.

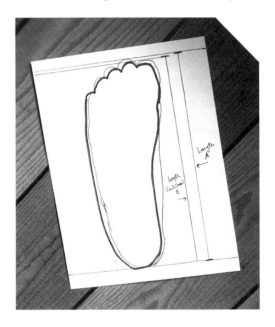

Try both of your feet and see how they compare. For example, my left "tricky hip" is chronically more internally rotated than my right when I'm not correcting it. The result is a longer, wider foot on the left. My left foot is more schmeared.

> I don't remember when I first was told I had flat feet, so I guess I assumed I was born with them. Progressively thicker and "more supportive" orthotics for my unusually flat feet did little to help my foot pain… or the knee, hip, and back pain I developed. When I developed horrible plantar fasciitis, enough was enough, and I went on a quest to fix my feet. Lo and behold, it was all schmear! [Your information] about foot schmear changed my feet and my life! I threw out my "supportive" footwear and started retraining and rehabilitating my poor feet (and legs). Fixing the foundation led to less knee and hip pain, and also a healthy obsession with alignment!
>
> AMANDA JOHNSON

MEASURING PRONATION CAN BE SLOPPY

Because the width of our feet and pelves (the plural of pelvis, which is pronounced PEL-vees and not a single-syllabled pelvz, which would be the little creatures that live in your pelvis and make cookies) are unique to each of us, the amount of displacement in each plane varies. If your pronation were measured via a simple data collection (i.e., considering only the inward displacement measure featured on page 37), but you had more rotation than you did translation, you might miss that your entire lower-body structure is operating off some of its axes. (Axes is the plural form of axis and is pronounced AX-ees.)

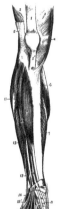

CHAPTER THREE

THE EARTH IS BUMPY

Speaking of shape, take a look at the stuff underneath your feet right now. I'll bet that over ninety percent of you are looking at flat and level ground. In fact, if you tallied up what's been under your feet your whole life, you'd find that most of it has been flat and level. Which means the parts of your body—the articulations and the muscle mass used via those articulations—that aren't required on flat and level surfaces have been lost. (And, P.S., flat and level would occur almost never in a natural environment, so not only do we have a particular foot and ankle shape created through this narrow, repetitive use, it's a *strange* shape at that.)

I'm hoping that by now you understand why the allopathic view of minimal shoes ("They cause injury!") is not entirely accurate, but also not without merit. And that the all-barefoot/minimal view ("It's natural!") is missing a key piece: your feet are not "natural" any longer, and neither is the stuff you walk on.

I once attended a lecture on barefoot living that was impressive in its inclusion of beautiful foot anatomy and force diagrams and explanations of how things work in the foot. I loved it. And I agreed entirely that being barefoot is necessary for optimal, whole-body function. But while the lecture was spot-on with the intra-foot physics, the forces listed for the foot did not include any outside of the foot. It was a "here's how the foot works" talk without any consideration given to the fact that the foot does not work in isolation. If you're going to use a biomechanics argument to support your recommendations, you have to use *all* of the mechanics—and include forces created by stepping with the foot.

SO, WHAT'S NATURAL?

❝ My feet grew a full size after starting to walk more barefoot and in minimal shoes. I can not fit in my first pair of Vibram Five Fingers from six years ago anymore. I can also do more pistol squats on one leg. I used to be able to do three or four, now I can do fifteen at a time. In the single-leg pistol squat, foot stability and proprioception are super important.

GALINA IVANOVA DENZEL

Think of the roots, rocks, mossy patches, and inclines of a forest floor. To walk (minimally shod or barefoot) across that surface requires literally countless joint angles and configurations as your feet adjust to each unique surface. The more inclines and declines on a walking surface, the more variation in ankle, knee, and hip use, pelvic positioning, and the greater variance in muscles used throughout the entire body. The more natural debris—twigs, leaves, mushrooms, stones—cluttering the surface, the more your whole-body musculature has to work. And, in both cases, the more of your "parts" you keep.

Now think of the sidewalks, roads, and indoor floors and walking tracks that your feet have spent a lifetime on. See the difference? Even if you've done a lot of walking in your lifetime, chances are most of it's been on unnaturally flat and level surfaces. And the hardness of concrete, while somewhat similar to the firmly packed dirt of a trail, still exceeds the natural biological forces created by the interface of natural on natural. The increase in impact, made worse by poor walking or running mechanics, can increase the risk of injuries like fractures.

One of the reasons I'm not barefoot all of the time is because I can't do it naturally. Shoes, one could argue, serve a role in buffering our bodies from a repetitive-use injury that could be made by the unnatural loads between the body and man-made ground, both in the case of its hardness and its flatness.

The body is tough and can handle the impact of walking on hard surfaces, but the repetition of doing so can cause injury, as every single step is an unnaturally high load. Can you just bend your knees to soften the blow to your feet? Sure you can.

DOCTOR'S NOTE

"As a podiatrist I'm constantly working with people to resolve or reduce the pain in their feet, but what I spend quite a bit of time doing in each appointment is illustrating how their foot position—and pressure on their 'sore spots'—is directly impacted by the position of their thigh bones.

Chronic internal rotation of the hip is a pronation creator. By learning more about the location of a neutral knee pit and working towards decreasing internal rotation, you can remove much of the pronation collapse. As for me, what I can do is put you into orthotics, designed to increase the position of the arch and control pronation, to change the loads. But this doesn't do too much for the problem of weakness in the hip and foot. I tell my patients they're going to have to do some work (via exercises and awareness) on their end for long-term success."

—Theresa Perales, DPM

That's why you have knees. But now you're compensating for the unnatural loads to the feet by creating unnatural loads to the knees.

By now you know it's not just your feet. Your hips' weakness, caused (in part) by the repetitive flatness of manmade surfaces (i.e., the lack of incline or decline) as well as your lack of walking in general, has resulted in your entire legs being off their axes. Which means your foot bones, soles of the feet, ankles, knees, and hips are oriented in a position that makes for wonky loads with every step.

So should I get rid of my shoes? Without getting rid of the habits (adaptations to shoes, sitting, little walking, walking on unnatural surfaces) that themselves create issues in my feet, I'm not so sure that's a good plan.

By walking on such artificial surfaces all of our lives, our amazing, strong, variable musculature has adapted, becoming very good at walking on one kind of ground. That sounds great, right? Adaptation is a good thing! In fact, adaptation isn't good or bad; adaptation is just adaptation. We have this idea that the body can endlessly adapt to whatever we choose to do, but that's not the case. We can adapt for a while, but there is always a biological tax. And in many cases, this tax is so far removed from the initial point of compensation, we don't even associate the two, which keeps us consuming the problematic load.

YOUR MISSION: MOBILIZE YOUR FEET, IN THE LAB AND ON THE FIELD

Many therapeutic modalities include joint stability exercises in the attempt to strengthen the ankles for handling detritus, walks over sand and stones, and rooty forest floors. But these exercises are typically done for just a few minutes a day; the rest of the time the client consumes the same mechanical environment—flat and level ground—while wearing shoes that prevent the parts within the foot from participating. Corrective exercises as a sole means to consume the "nutritious loads" necessary for whole-body function require off-roading. While flat-ground walking is a great way to get some of you in shape, not all of you is getting healthier for the effort. So, like supplementing your diet with vitamin B12, you're going to have to supplement your walking with actual over-ground walking. You're going to have to start walking—on the actual ground, in as many forms as you can find.

A huge part of transitioning to minimal footwear is working to un-adapt our feet (and the rest of our bodies) away from the artificial environments to which they've been exposed. Your strong around-town feet aren't necessarily suited for all-terrain walking, and in order to reap the benefits of the dips and hills and lumps and bumps found in nature, your feet have to be supple enough to allow these movements. Mobilizing exercises might seem very passive, but they can be the most difficult, because our feet have been in casts for most of our lives and getting them to move can be a bit painful. I'll help you break down the loads to keep the stress on your feet gradual and your foot-restoration program rolling along.

By this point, you know that the health of your feet isn't dependent on your feet alone. Your feet are affected by what your whole body is doing (and vice versa), including what you put on your feet. A whole-body problem demands whole-body solutions. The good news is, you'll find your new to-do list waiting for you on the following pages. Have fun!

GENERAL GUIDELINES FOR FOOTWEAR TRANSITION

Here are some general guidelines to keep in mind as you transition from more supportive shoes to more supportive feet and from moving less to moving more.

Give underutilized muscle time to develop via corrective exercises. Begin foot exercises before switching shoes, and continue the foot exercises while doing your whole-body training in less supportive shoes.

Master shoeless walking before you try shoeless running. Running creates greater forces in the joints of the foot, so walking is the more natural precursor to developing the appropriate strength for running. Before you run five or eight miles in minimal shoes, make sure you've walked five or eight continuous, well-paced miles in them first.

Once you're ready for running, start with short distances first—on dirt or grass—before logging longer runs.

Seek out expert guidance on walking and running form. Conventional running shoes offer excessive cushioning to protect against high joint forces. The better you align your feet (and your body above your feet) while exercising, the less you will overload them.

MOVE

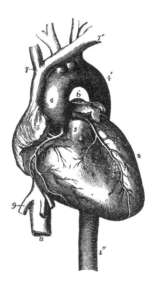

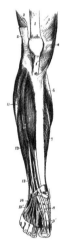

CHAPTER FOUR

STANCE HABITS TO CHANGE

If I asked you, "How much do you weigh?" you'd hop onto a scale and tell me the number that it gives you. But that number is really how much all of you weighs when you're standing on the scale. If you had a tiny scale in each knee, you could get them to give different numbers just by putting more of "your weight" over one foot. How you stand matters when it comes to loads in the body.

Right now you have a way of standing that is based on your movement history, including the kind of shoes you have worn. Just because you take your shoes off doesn't mean you'll automatically stand differently. Well, you will stand differently right away, but it might not be differently enough—especially if you're motivated by musculoskeletal pain.

The following are general guidelines on how to balance your weight evenly over and between your feet, as well as how to position your feet relative to your knees and hips, and how to carry your weight relative to the ground, to allow more of your body to participate in standing and moving. In the long term, a new stance can lead to more stability of your body parts, which can lead to improved health.

Because you're likely to be using your body outside of "doing your exercises" and because your body is adapting to inputs one hundred percent of the time, adjusting your habitual stance can have an even greater impact than just doing exercise. When you adjust your posture you're essentially doing the same thing as an exercise—creating a new load and asking your body to adapt. For best results put your exercises on a calendar and stick to them, and keep these stance modifications in the front of your mind, ensuring constant adjustments all day long.

If you're standing around—and you're often going to be standing around—constantly cycle through the following list of adjustments to balance out your loads.

START STRAIGHTENING YOUR FEET

While we all have different movement backgrounds, a shared cultural theme (flat ground, shoes, sitting the bulk of the day starting as five- or six-year-olds) seems to have resulted in a similar adaptation: most of us tend to stand, walk, and run with our feet splayed outward to varying degrees. Because the position of the foot sets the stage for the way the joint axes and muscles line up from the toes to the hip, the feet need to be brought forward to maximize leverage.

Find your best "feet forward" by aligning the outer edges of each foot using the points shown in the pic: the bony prominence just behind the little toe and the other a spot on the foot found by dropping an imaginary vertical line from the outer ankle bone to the floor.

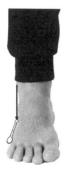 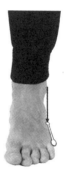

No, it's not necessary to force your body all the way straight right off the bat; there are many tissues that need to adapt to this new position. However, your exercises should all use this baseline as much as possible. And when you're walking, you can attempt to correct to whatever degree suits you.

And I'm compelled to say that keeping your feet straight is really much more complicated than I'm making it seem here, but I want you to have an idea of where we're headed. For a more nuanced and complex look at how to keep your feet straight, see Chapter Ten: Fix Your Feet All Day.

WHOLE BODY BAREFOOT

FEET PELVIS-WIDTH APART

As I mentioned at the beginning of this section, the weight (weight isn't the ultimately correct term here, but I think it's the easiest to understand and therefore I'm using it, mmkay?) that gets placed on the joints depends on how the bones and muscles line up. For many of us, the way the foot-knee-hip line stacks up results in a higher-than-normal load on the medial (towards the midline) side of the knee, which is a risk factor for ACL (anterior cruciate ligament) and medial meniscus tears.

To reduce medial loads when standing or walking, try this:

Standing in front of a mirror, line up the middle of the front of your ankles with the bony prominences at the front of your pelvis. (This better distributes the weight of the body over the entirety of both knees. This arrangement is easier to do when standing than while walking, but even widening your ankles slightly makes a difference. If, for example, you tend to walk with your ankles very close together—similar to walking on a tightrope—open them just a bit, bringing the ankles closer to pelvis-width apart.

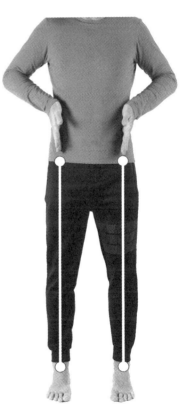

Another way to check this "line up" is to go up and down stairs. After planting your foot on the stair, does your knee end up dropping inwards as you transfer your weight onto it?

All of these scenarios—close-footed walking, inward knee dropping, and standing with your ankles too far apart or too close together—make for wonky knee loads. And the wider the pelvis, the greater the medial knee loads with narrow foot placement. This is likely one of the reasons women struggle more with ACL issues and knee osteoarthritis.

BACK YOUR HIPS UP

If you stand sideways to a mirror and hang a plumb line down from the center of your hip joint, you'll probably find that the other end is dangling over the front of your foot.

The loads created by standing this way are problematic for many reasons, but setting aside things like increased psoas tension, lower-back compression, and reduced weight-bearing status of the hips, it's also a big problem for your feet.

If you find that you do tend to stand with your pelvis out in front of you—a totally normal adaptation to wearing heeled shoes for your entire life—then the bulk of your weight is being carried over the small bones of your feet, instead of being distributed throughout larger, stronger bones in the shins, ankles, and heels. Pelvic thrust also makes it difficult to rotate your thighs (the next stop on the alignment train) because your quads have to tighten to keep your whole body from pitching forward.

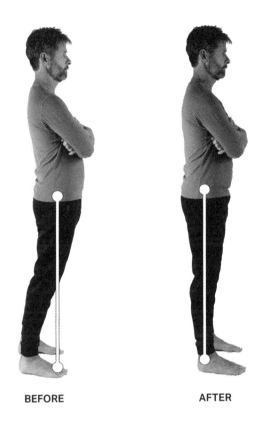

BEFORE   **AFTER**

To correct pelvic thrust, move your hips back so that they're directly over the knees and ankles—so that the plumb line picks up the midpoint of the knee and the quarter-sized ankle bone over the heel.

Now your large heel bone is bearing the weight of your body above it, reducing the pressure on the front of the feet (and any nerves, neuromas, or hypermobile toe joints that are in there). This allows your feet the freedom they need to be dexterous, and helps release the quads so the thigh bones are free to move.

NEUTRAL FEMURS

Now it's time to *unschmear*.

First, bend your knees a few times, feeling for the hamstring tendons behind the knee as you do. Second, stand with a mirror behind you to look for the indentations these tendons make on the backs of your knees (an area I call "knee pits").

Then, standing, feet straight and weight back over your heels, with a mirror or a close friend behind you for guidance, rotate your thighs until these indentations line up directly behind you.

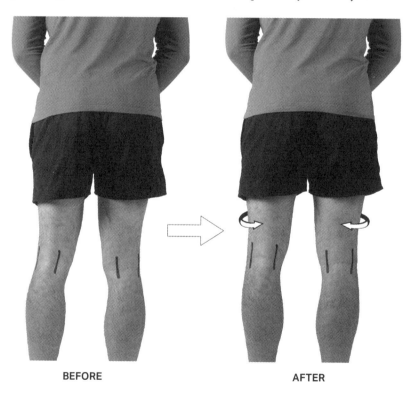

BEFORE   AFTER

Lining up your knee pits and your feet at the same time will undo any schmear while you're standing and it will also create an immediate arch, even in those who are otherwise "flat-footed."

Note that the degree to which you need to rotate your femurs will depend on how much they've been rotated, and will probably vary between your two legs. Also important to note: you do NOT need to keep the instep of the foot down as you rotate your knee pits to neutral. To do so can torque the knee, so let the inner edges of the feet lift away from the ground! Eventually they'll be able to stay on the ground when your knee is in neutral, but that will take lots of the intrinsic foot muscle mobilization exercises in the next section.

All habits can be difficult to change, either mentally or physically. As far as overcoming the mental hump, strive to keep the stance points in mind as you move through your day.

As far as physical difficulty goes, the following is a list of corrective exercises designed to mobilize the typically underused parts of your body and restore lost ranges of motion and muscle so you can move better. You should find that the exercises done in conjunction with the all-day alignment awareness reinforce each other. Meaning, it will become easier to "get into position" when necessary, and by doing so with regularity, the need for the correctives will decrease. Your body will become mobile simply from the way you use it in day-to-day life.

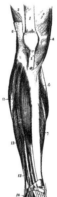

CHAPTER FIVE

STRETCHING THE INTRINSIC TISSUES OF THE FOOT

Intrinsic foot muscles are those that both start and end within the foot, and in this section I'm including all "musculoskel-etal" tissues—bone, ligament, tendon, and fascia—that reside within the foot alone. Because your foot has been contained in a shoe for the bulk of your life, chances are you haven't been walking on surfaces that would naturally be pushing the tiny bones in your feet around—which is unfortunate, as it is that passive deformation that results in the muscles responding and adapting to these movements.

The flexible, thin sole of minimal footwear will let a lot of this motion in now, but your feet have essentially been casted for decades. In the same way I wouldn't recommend ripping off an arm cast and doing a hundred pushups, I don't recommend throwing your ill-prepared feet into nature.

With a lack of muscle use comes less circulation (read: nourishment) to all the tissues of the feet—including bone. Research into minimally shod running has shown an increase in bone marrow edema—the precursor for bone fractures. Why? Who knows. Form, level of impact, hardness of ground, distances traveled, and health of the foot tissue to begin with are all players in the equation that is Your Foot Injury. What I do know is that most people I know have spent decades *not* loading their intrinsic foot tissues, and most people coming to me with foot injuries have difficulty recruiting the fine motor skills that should be inherent to feet. So let's start there.

PASSIVE TOE SPREADING

Separating—also known as abducting—your toes mobilizes the bones, muscles, and connective tissues in your feet so you can start achieving better intrinsic muscle strength, circulation, and nerve health. Eventually you will be doing this with the muscles within the feet, but first you'll start by using the muscles of your hands.

Start by sitting with one ankle crossed over the opposite knee. With your hands, gently spread your toes apart, stretching the toes away from each other. Ideally you'll hold the toes apart for a minute at a time, but start with smaller distances and shorter intervals—maybe fifteen seconds—and progress to greater distances and longer holds as you feel comfortable.

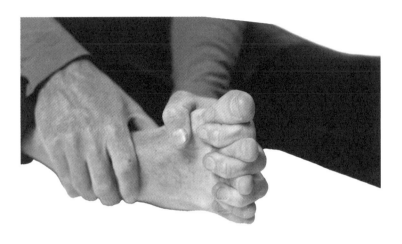

Eventually you can interlace your fingers and toes together—the same way you would with your hands, but with one hand and one foot instead. I like to hang out like this when I'm reading or watching movies. Bonus: you'll end up doing some hip stretching as well because WHO PUT MY FEET SO FAR AWAY?

If you've read my other books/blog posts, you know I'm all about time management and getting movement done while you're doing other things. You might have four hours to spend pulling your toes apart (which sounds like a lot, but I'd bet you've never balked once at your shoes pressing them together ten hours a day, every day for the last thirty years), but then again probably you don't. Easy solution: get some toe-alignment products like toe-spreading socks and toe-spacers. This makes a passive stretch even *more* passive—you don't even need your hands. Yes, I said it. Hands-free foot health is available, if you want it.

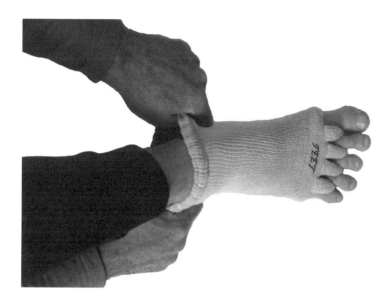

Wear your spacers/socks overnight or while you watch TV so that you'll be working your foot kinks out while getting something else done. Like sleeping. (For what it's worth, I woke up three hours into the first night sleeping with my alignment socks on. My feet were screaming—they had had enough exercise for one night. Listen to your body!)

STANDING FOOT MASSAGE

So you've got your thighs in neutral but the ball of your foot is miles from the ground. Why? In general, the thirty-three joints of the foot have lost all their mobility—they've clumped together as a response to negative input (the surfaces and shoes you have walked upon didn't require that these joints stay mobile) and now your "foot" motion comes only from the ankle. Want evenly mobile feet? Start introducing low and controlled loads to the feet that will mobilize the muscles and joints within them.

Start standing with a tennis or similarly sized squishy ball under the arch of one foot. Slowly load your weight onto the ball, moving your foot forward and back and side to side to apply pressure to individual joints within the foot.

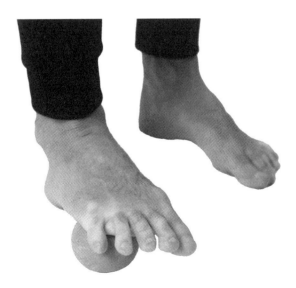

I told you that there were thirty-three joints in each foot already, yes? Well, I'm telling you again. Think of your foot as a floor you must vacuum. When it's your turn to vacuum, you don't just go around the edges, do you? Vacuum along a single line down the arch of the floor? Nope, you vacuum all of it. Apply this diligence to your foot massage. Move tiny distances at a time. Leave no foot joint unstimulated. (Note: Again, if you live in a vacuum, this does not pertain to you, as why would you ever be vacuuming?)

Work the sole of the foot with the ball, applying more or less pressure as needed. Eventually try different ball sizes and firmnesses. Each will mobilize the joints differently.

“ I come from a family of bunion-makers. They all wear orthotics as well. By age twenty I also was the proud owner of my own orthotics, and debilitating back pain. By thirty I realized this just wasn't working. I ditched the orthotics, started going barefoot, started stretching my feet. By thirty-five I was doing lots of yoga and wearing the most flexible shoes I could find, by forty-four I found you online, and realized “I'm on the right track.” Here I am at forty-eight, cruising through the first level of your course, learning even more, getting stronger, and I have no bunions!”

ALIX RODRIGUES

TOP OF THE FOOT STRETCH

This stretch is great for undoing chronic "gripping" tension in the toes and the front of the ankle. Refer back to the "what your feet do in flip-flops" graphic to see how this stretch undoes the specific motions necessary to keep on an unattached shoe. If you're a chronic flip-flop wearer, then this exercise is especially pertinent to *your* feet.

Holding on to something if necessary, stand on your right foot and reach your left foot back behind you, tucking the toes of your left foot under and placing them on the floor.

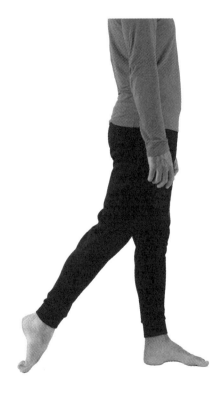

The tendency here is to lean the entire body forward to reduce the load to the feet. If your body is really leaning forward, then shorten the distance you've reached the leg back or sit down in a chair to lessen the load.

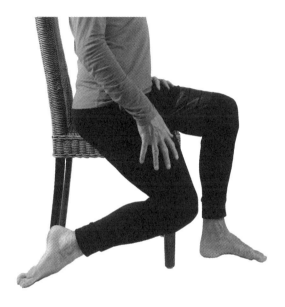

Once you're used to the load, try bringing your pelvis over your standing (not your stretching) ankle, and try to bring the upper body over the hips. Once here you can decrease the stretch by bringing your left foot forward, closer to your right foot, or increase it by moving it farther back.

The goal is to work up to holding this stretch for a minute, but it's very common to experience cramping. If you do, just come out of the stretch, wait till the cramp passes, then try again. And then, of course, switch feet.

This is a super portable stretch that you can do any time you're standing. Do it a few times every day until your feet regain their intended dexterity and/or until you've eliminated any cramping.

The Top of the Foot Stretch targets not only intrinsic foot muscles, but extrinsic ones as well, which makes it the perfect segue into…

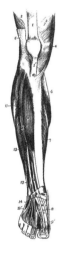

CHAPTER SIX

STRETCHING THE EXTRINSIC TISSUES OF THE FOOT

Extrinsic foot muscles are those that have one attachment in the foot and one outside of it. Basically anything that passes over the ankle, moving the foot relative to the shin or thigh, counts as an extrinsic foot tissue, and as you work on these, you'll see how footwear really does create whole-body alignment problems.

CALF STRETCH – GASTROCNEMIUS

I often say that if I could make everyone do just one stretch, it would be this one. There are a few reasons for this. The first is that our calf muscles are chronically shortened in this culture due to heeled shoes (which create forced plantarflexion, a.k.a. toe-pointing) and sitting (forced calf shortening via knee flexion). If you've worn shoes and sat throughout your life, you're missing an essential distribution of mass. Second, your calf muscles have some of the greatest responsibilities when it comes to keeping you upright and mobile. Critical for the endurance of standing and controlled walking (which is the opposite of "walking is falling"), you need your calves to be in tip-top shape. And thirdly (but not finally; I could go on and on, but I won't, this one time), the tension in your lower body while walking has a whip-like effect on the top. Meaning your upper spine and head can be unduly accelerated by tension IN YOUR CALVES.

Have you ever seen a wave break? Well, here's how it works. A section of water comes to shore at the same speed. But as a wave approaches shallow water, the inclined sea bed slows the bottom of the wave down, causing the upper part of the wave to accelerate right on over. And so, it breaks.

Now picture a gait pattern where the lower part of the leg is slowed down due to tension between the foot and the shin. What happens? The shin is slowed down relative to the whole body, accelerating the upper body over the slowed bottom half. No biggie, since you can compensate by simultaneously firing opposing muscles to keep that forward motion from happening (i.e. you can prevent a net forward motion), but what you end up with is a walking pattern that tenses your upper back and neck with every step. This way of firing your muscles can result in chronically tensed muscles down the back of the neck, shoulders, and upper spine—muscles that have adapted to the tension in your leg.

Why is this important, you ask? If you're working on neck and shoulder issues, wondering why they're not getting better, consider that these parts need to stay tense to cope with the forces created by HOW YOU WALK.

And now, the calf stretches.

Place the ball of your left foot on the apex of a half-foam roller (I use a 6 x 3 x 12-inch one) or a rolled-up folded towel, drop the heel all the way to the ground, and straighten that knee. Hang out here for a bit, then try to step forward with your right foot.

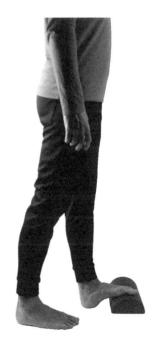
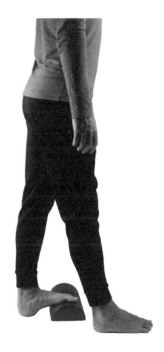

You should be able to bring your right foot all the way forward, but most people can't do this immediately. Instead, take a smaller step—your right foot might remain behind your left, or be at the same level, or only a little bit forward. Keep your weight stacked vertically over the heel of whichever foot is farther back.

You can make this stretch easier by bringing the front leg back a little bit, or by sliding the foot on the roller back a little bit to keep the toes lower. If you're really struggling—say you're having trouble standing upright, or you have to tense your whole body to keep the tension in your lower leg from launching your body off the dome—ditch the foam roller. Start with a folded-then-rolled towel or the front of a phone book, which both tend to be shorter than the dome. You can move back to the dome after you've mobilized some of the tissues in your lower leg.

Stretch the calf muscles in both legs as many times in a day as you can, for up to a minute at a time. I like to leave a half-foam roller in a few different rooms of the house so I can stretch my calves while I'm on the phone, brushing my teeth, or making supper.

This stretch targets the gastrocnemius muscle.

CALF STRETCH – SOLEUS

This stretch is a companion to the above Calf Stretch, targeting the soleus (which is the deeper muscle of the calf) and the Achilles tendon, both of which are shorter than necessary in most of us.

Place the ball of your right foot on top of the dome or rolled towel again, and lower your heel to the floor. Step forward until your left foot is even with or a little in front of the right, and then bend your right knee without lifting your heel (your other knee can bend too). Hold this for thirty to sixty seconds, and repeat on the left side.

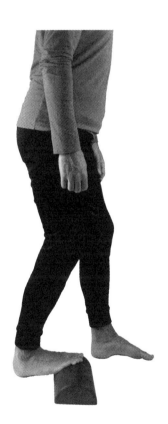

The soleus is often neglected in a calf-stretching regimen because it requires a different joint configuration than what's necessary for targeting the other calf muscles in the group. How much do you need this one? As much as all the others, so make sure to do this stretch as often as you do the other Calf Stretch.

> " Minimal shoes have eliminated my plantar fasciitis, which I had for a year or so. It kept getting worse, until I dropped the overbuilt shoes and started lowering my heels and going barefoot. Over a year, I went from cross trainers to Nike Frees to flat soles. Now, any shoe with a traditional heel and arch support leaves my feet aching and tired. It's been almost six years and my plantar fasciitis has not returned."
>
> *ROLAND DENZEL*

DOUBLE CALF STRETCH

This stretch continues the work of the Calf Stretch, but also targets the hamstrings and connective tissues (fasciae) that wrap around the series of joints that make up the feet and leg. I know that the hamstrings may seem super far (seventeen inches) from your feet, but, like, everything's connected, man. Tight hamstrings keep the knees slightly buckled, which in turn keeps the calves and Achilles tendons short—OR IS IT THE OTHER WAY AROUND? One can't really say. Either way, this stretch helps you recognize the adaptations that come about from sitting and standing, and slowly nudges these tissues into a different state.

Stand in front of a chair, facing the seat. With your feet pelvis-width apart, knees straight, and feet pointing forward, tip the pelvis forward until your palms rest on the chair.

Can't reach the chair without really bending the knees or rounding the back?

Stop! and make your seat height higher or move to a counter or desk top.

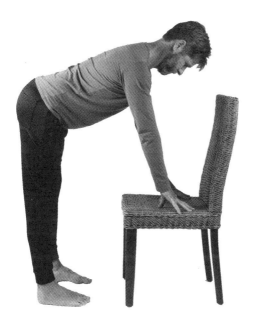

Once your arms are down, see if you can allow your spine to drop down toward the floor, and your tailbone to lift toward the ceiling. Don't force your ribs to the floor or arch your back—just consciously *relax* the spine to the ground as much as you can.

If you noticed your back was curved upward like an angry cat, it means that the tension down the back of the leg is there, all the time, working on your spine, knees, or both. If you can pepper your day with this stretch (makes for a great break from sitting), you'll notice an improvement.

Other pointers on this one include:

Keep your weight back in your heels, far enough back that you can wiggle your toes. Relax the back of your neck. Really. Try lowering the top of your head toward the ground, which moves the load into the fascial wrapping extending down your entire backside.

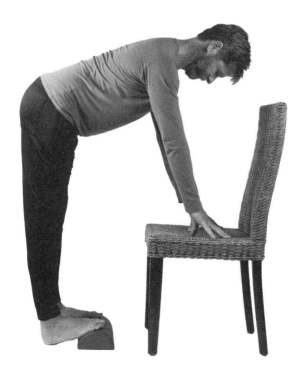

WHOLE BODY BAREFOOT

Once you can hold this for sixty seconds comfortably, add your half-foam roller or rolled towel in front of the chair, and repeat the stretch with the balls of the feet on the apex of the roller.

This ups the ante quite a bit. Add it when you feel ready.

STRAP STRETCH

This stretch focuses on connecting, for the exerciser, the relationship between tension in the calf and coping mechanisms like bending the knees and pointing the toes.

Lie on your back and loop a strap (or a belt) across the toe-box of your right foot. Straighten your right leg above you and extend your left leg until your left hamstring is touching the floor. If you have to bring your right leg lower for the left hamstring to touch, do so, keeping both legs straight. Allow your arms to hold the weight of your right leg—relax it completely.

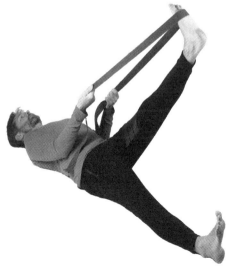

Now, pull your foot toward you—with the strap, not with the muscles down the front of the shin. Keeping your ankle in place, pull your right leg higher in small increments, without allowing the left hamstring to come up off the floor. You might notice that, in order to reduce the stretch to these areas, you'll want to point the toes slightly or bend the knee. This is a normal reaction, but it's also what allows the tension down the back of the leg—and the resulting gait patterns from this tension—to persist. The goal is not a huge, uncomfortable stretch, but a gentle stretching load to muscles that very much want to avoid it.

After you have held this for a while, bring your right leg across the body and hold the stretch there (which introduces new loads to the hip muscles that help you walk with a wider stance).

Do this one a lot. Bonus: You have to get down on the floor and back up again so it's got other necessary movement "nutrients" in it as well. Strap Stretch is *floortified* with movement nutrition. Get it?

CATSUIT STRETCH

Before you do this next exercise, I'd like you to put yourself in an imaginary outfit—one that wraps your body head-to-toe and is skintight. Are you wearing it in your mind? Great. Are you wearing it in real life? Quick, go get your camera and send me a picture immediately, thanks.

Now that you're in your imaginary suit, imagine how that suit would wrinkle or gather as your body changed the orientation of parts from neutral to sitting in a chair or wearing heeled shoes. You see, when the pelvis thrusts, or the chest lifts, the ankles plantarflex, the knees bend, etc., it doesn't only require the re-arrangement of bones. These motions require the rearrangement of the tissue wrappings *over* the bones and muscles as well.

In general, the way most people's imaginary catsuits have adjusted to the backward "fixing" of the forward projection created by heeled shoes is by shortening areas of the suit on the backside and lengthening the suit on the front.

Again, this phenomenon is not local to the ankles, but includes "suit wrinkles" all the way up to the back of the neck. The neck! From what's on your feet!

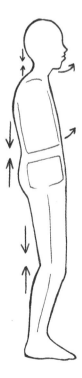

So you can see why foot issues are really whole-body issues. Which is why this next stretch targets both the muscles and the connective tissues all along the back line of the body.

Sit on the floor with your feet pressed flat against a wall and your legs straight.

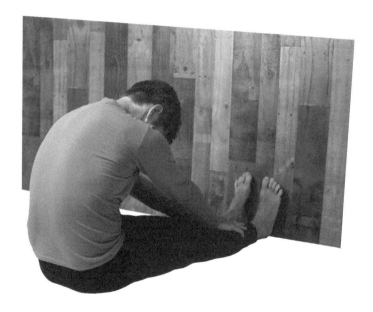

If this is difficult for you because your hamstrings are too tight—if your pelvis is being forced to tuck backwards, straining your lower back (see above)—feel free to sit your bottom up on as many pillows as you need to be comfortable (image right).

Fold your body forward, tipping your pelvis towards the wall as you drop your chest towards your legs. Don't force it, just drop

WHOLE BODY BAREFOOT

to wherever you can get to using gravity alone. Now, completely relax your neck, letting your head hang. Feel how the motion of your head creates an additional pull down the back of your legs? Maybe you can feel how your tendency to jut your chin up and toward the computer all day is "connected" to your lower back?

This exercise is one of my favorites because it helps people experience how, indeed, everything can be connected: your head position to the position of your sacrum, your shoe choices to chronic neck issues.

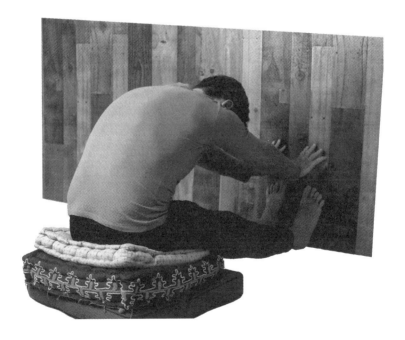

MOVE YOUR NOOKS AND CRANNIES

Sometimes it takes more than exercises to get the smaller areas of the body moving. Bodywork can be helpful in finding the areas of your body that don't move, but sometimes you can move some of your in-between spaces yourself, using tools designed to fit gently into sedentary areas.

The lower legs are incredibly complex in the movements they can create. Below, Jill Miller, fascia expert and yoga therapist, shares additional ways to help you move the muscles of your lower leg even more.

CALF STACK by Jill Miller, author of *The Roll Model®: A Step-by-Step Guide to Erase Pain, Improve Mobility, and Live Better in Your Body*

Calf Stack

Calf Stack is a category of moves where you use two Yoga Tune Up (or other) balls, one on either side of your calf, to increase the slide and glide of the dense myofascial tissue in your lower leg.

In every stack (see different options in the next two pages), the balls are placed to simultaneously nuzzle into the right and left side of your shin (if you've got your anatomy book handy, one ball goes along the anterior tibialis and the other along the peroneal group) as you apply pressure.

In all stacks, once you've set up the move, point, flex, and circle your ankle and foot, then re-stack the balls higher or lower along your lower leg and repeat. Spend five to ten minutes per leg.

STACK 1

Sitting on the floor or a cushion in whatever way you can, bring one bent leg in front of your body, placing a ball beneath the outside of your shin. Stack a second ball on top and hold in place with your hand.

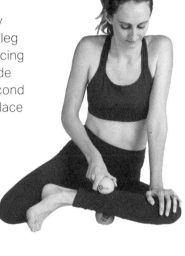

STACK 2

Sitting on the floor or a cushion, position your lower leg on top of one ball on the floor. Then cross your other leg over the top to sandwich a second ball between your two legs.

STACK 3

Lie on your side with a pillow beneath your head, hips and knees bent to 90°. Stack one ball on the floor under your first leg, then stack a second ball on top, pinning it with a block and your other leg on top.

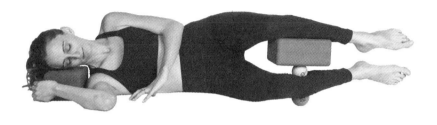

WHOLE BODY BAREFOOT

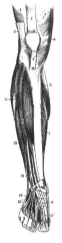

STRENGTHENING THE INTRINSIC TISSUES OF THE FOOT

TOE ABDUCTION

The term *abduct* as used in anatomy means "to take away from the midline." This is a very simple way to both test and improve the health of your foot musculature.

Stand with your feet pelvis-width apart and pointing straight ahead, and your weight back in your heels. Now try to spread your toes apart as far as you can, just like you can spread your fingers. Try to make space between each toe, keeping all the toes flat on the ground (image next page).

Not surprising, but many chronically shod folks have lost their ability to abduct their toes—a lifetime of shoes that push your toes together has rendered your toes almost unresponsive to your brain's signals…at first. The good news is that the more you try to do this exercise in conjunction with the manual/passive toe-spreading, the better your toes will respond to the signals you're sending.

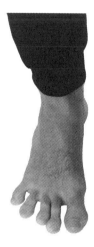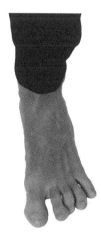

Repeat this exercise throughout the day, with or without shoes (and you'll know whether your shoes are too tight in the toe-box if you can't do this exercise in them).

This is one of the first exercises I give not only to those interested in transitioning to minimal shoes, but also to those wanting better balance, foot-nerve health, and better functioning knees and hips.

TOE LIFTS

Once you've tested your ability to spread or splay your toes, how about seeing if you can lift them…one at a time? I know, I know. Toes seem so small and light. But in this exercise they can feel heavy.

Try to lift just your big toes while in the same stance as the last exercise. Try the right foot, then the left. Most of us can lift all our toes at once, but find it difficult to use the muscles separately.

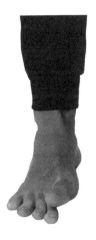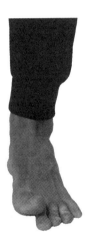

The muscle group working to lift your big toe (the extensor hallucis group) is one of the strongest muscles in the foot. Getting these muscles working can go a long way toward restoring strength and motor control in your feet, crucial for stabilized motions at the ankle, knee, and hip. (Again, IT'S ALL

CONNECTED.) Work to lift each big toe straight upward, rather than letting it veer sideways (toward the pinkie toe).

After you've mastered lifting your big toes try lifting first them and then the second toe of each foot, making sure to keep the balls of your feet on the floor. Then lift the third, fourth, and fifth toes. Once all the toes are lifted, put them back down one by one. Then try this again, but one foot at a time.

When you're finished, stretch your toes with the Top of the Foot Stretch—it's common to feel cramping in the arch during this exercise, since these muscles have rarely if ever been used before.

> " Three years ago I was prescribed orthotics to help me with my hammertoe. During three months of problems with the orthotics, I kept thinking that this wasn't natural and there had to be a better way. Enter Katy. My sister had come across her blog. It made total sense. Two-plus years later, I have no foot pain and my hammertoe has become quite flexible. "
>
> CHRISTINE PILGER

CHAPTER EIGHT

STRENGTHENING THE EXTRINSIC TISSUES OF THE FOOT

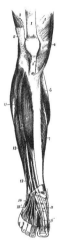

The following exercises target the muscles between the foot and the rest of the body, specifically how these muscles are moving during the functional task of *being upright and walking around safely*. Walking—as boring as it sounds—can quickly become something you cannot do. Whether this is due to foot pain, knee injury, osteoarthritis, or just a lack of strength, losing the ability to walk is a profound weight on the mind. You're probably a great walker, but take it from me—taking it from thousands of others I've been in direct contact with: Keep your walking skills up, because you'll surely miss them when they go.

SINGLE-LEG BALANCE

Balance is one of those things rarely thought about until after a fall. And I think many people operate under the assumption that they have pretty good balance, even though they've hardly tested their skills. In reality, most of us might have had great balance at one time, but since we aren't regularly exposed to balance challenges, we're comfortable in our abilities until we end up on the ground, wondering what knocked us over.

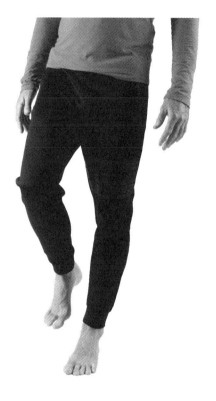

Test yourself. Barefoot, and standing on a flat surface, stand on the left leg with the knee straight (but not hyperextended) and bend the right knee to lift the right foot slightly off the floor. What's your ankle doing? Your arms? Shoulders? How about your face? Was that grimace there before you got started? Now, check the position of your standing foot. Did it turn out, pointing slightly to the right or left? What about your standing knee? Did it automatically bend to lower your center of mass, reducing the work to the hip?

　　　　　　　　　　　WHOLE BODY BAREFOOT

Whatever you did, take note of how your body structurally rearranges itself to deal with balance. Then, consider that every walking step requires a period of balance and that what you do to cope—bend the knees, turn out the feet, reach your arms out to the sides—is slowly creeping into your gait pattern until, eventually, your ability to walk with balance is all the way gone and you've become a shuffler.

Try this exercise again, this time keeping your ankle still, your arms down by your sides, and your foot pointing straight ahead (with knee pits facing back, once you're more advanced). This ensures you're training your leg as it is best used in a level-ground gait, and assists in targeting more use of the lateral hip muscles responsible for correcting schmear. Hold this for up to a minute on each side, three times each.

It's normal to think that one day you get old and, surprise! your ability to do stuff is gone. But in most cases, you've stopped doing a movement for a long time, the muscles and programming necessary to do it have atrophied, and when you call on the move, it's gone. Continue to keep up your balance work—you'll be glad you did!

SINGLE-LEG TOWEL BALANCE

This exercise takes the previous one up a notch and is a necessary step to prepare the body for walking on more varied terrain—the instability of the towel will deepen the work in the foot, ankle, thigh, and hip muscles.

Fold a towel over several times and repeat the single-leg

balance while standing on top of the towel, balancing for up to one minute before switching legs. To make this even more challenging, turn your head from side to side to mix up your visual field. Want to really up the ante? Try it with your eyes closed.

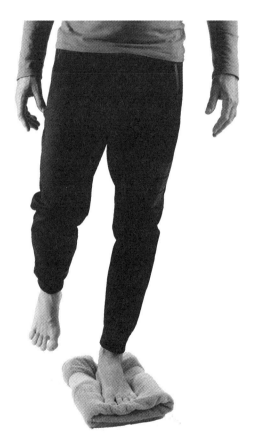

PELVIC LIST

This exercise might seem very similar to the previous two, but the List demands isolated work from your lateral hip muscles and is perhaps the best schmear-buster of all, when done with a neutral knee-pit (which is an advanced move, so give yourself time). Standing in neutral—feet straight, ankles pelvis-width apart, weight on the rear of the foot—place your right hand on your right hip and pull the right side of the pelvis down toward the floor. Bringing the right half of the pelvis down lifts the left half up and will result in your left foot clearing the ground. Neither knee bends during this exercise, and you'll want to make sure you're not using the muscles in your lower back to hike the left hip up—a common "cheat."

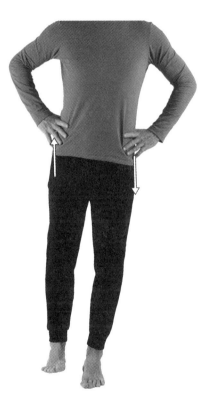

If you feel your standing ankle wobble, touch your left foot down by pointing your toes or hold on to a chair or wall. If you feel the need to move your weight forward over the front of your right foot again or notice your knees are bending, these are signs that you don't regularly use your lateral hip muscles when walking. And you probably have some significant schmear going on. Try working on holding this for up to a minute, three times on each side.

NEXT-LEVEL LIST

Once you've incorporated the Pelvic List and other exercises and habits into your daily routine, try advancing the List while standing on a phone book or yoga block with the other leg floating above the ground. You'll follow the same listing procedure, but in addition to the pelvis hiking up, you can lower the floating half of the pelvis down, increasing the lateral hip muscles' working range of motion. Controlled motion over a greater range of motion will better prepare these muscles— and you—for going up and down hills, which you're going to be doing a lot once you're done with this book, right?

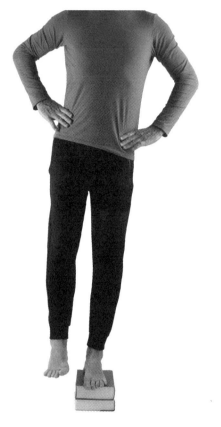

WHOLE BODY BAREFOOT

NEXT-NEXT LEVEL LIST

If you've been trying to list with a neutral knee pit, you've probably noticed how challenging it is. Mostly because by the time you rotate your thighs to neutral, the entire instep of the foot is off the ground. How can you stand on the outside of your foot and list at the same time? The answer is, you can't. But here's a trick: stand on an inverted half-foam roller (flat side up, round side down).

By doing so, you'll bring the "floor" (that is, the flat side of the dome) over to match the angle of your foot. By taking your foot's limitations out of the equation, you'll be using all of your listing muscles!

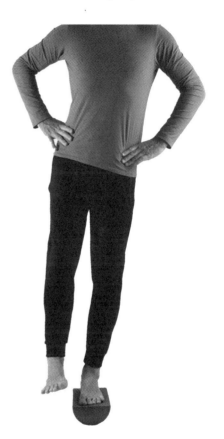

CALF ELEVATORS

The calf muscles are the elevators of the body. Lifting and lowering the body to and from the ground, the calf muscles really come into play with varied terrain. Unfortunately, void of a well-rounded environment, our calves have lost the ability to work in their primary plane of action—straight up and down. Instead of a stable ankle when moving this part, "up and down" now includes elements of rotation and sideways motion (image below left).

Try a calf raise and notice, when you come up onto your toes, does one or both of your ankles move away from each other? Do you roll onto the outside of the foot? Maybe your heels come closer together?

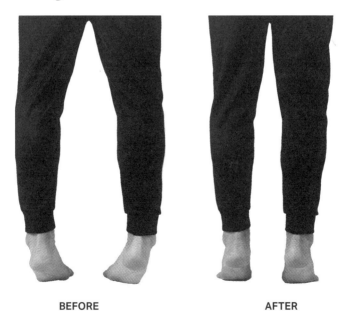

BEFORE   **AFTER**

This type of calf raise isn't really the plantarflexion/dorsiflexion action stable ankles depend on. And I don't know about you, but when I take an elevator I want it to go straight up or down, not sideways, or in a circle. Unstable ankles in a calf raise are unstable ankles when you're walking, running, or hiking, which is why I suggest swapping Calf Raises for Calf Elevators.

Calf Elevators are a great way to isolate those calf and foot muscles that aren't working and help develop a better-supported multi-terrain gait pattern.

Standing in front of a mirror, line up your feet so they point forward, ankles pelvis-width apart. Pressing the front of your foot into the ground, slowly lift your heels away from the ground without shoving your pelvis forward. (P.S. Shoving your pelvis forward is a great way to use momentum to get up instead of using your calf muscles.) While going up and down, keep your ankles straight—imagine a pin going through both ankles, keeping them fixed both relative to the ground and relative to each other. Keep the instep of the foot reaching down towards the floor, keep the ball of the foot on the floor, and make sure you're not on your toes. Your toes should be lift-able throughout the entire exercise (image page 102, right).

Initially you can do this holding on to something, but eventually you should do elevator (straight up and down) calf raises without holding on to anything. You don't have a wall or chair there when you're hiking, so it's best to not train yourself to require balancing items while walking.

Eventually (once you can "elevator" with both ankles stable), try it one leg at a time. Moving uphill requires that you be able to stabilize the ankle while propelling your body upward—one step at a time. To neglect to train each ankle to hold your entire body weight is to be half-prepared for the "athletic pursuit" of walking uphill.

“ At fifty-two years of age, I'd suffered from foot pain for decades. At shoe stores, I'd try on thirty pairs of shoes, going for comfort over style, and walk out with nothing because they all hurt my feet. Three different pairs of custom-made orthotics over the years, stick-on metatarsal pads, tens of pairs of the most popular shoes with contoured insoles, overly padded running shoes, the typical nurses' shoes, and physical therapy all left me worse off than when I started. Last spring I found [your exercises] at the library and they changed my life. I took off my shoes, got the whole DVD series with half-domes, yoga blocks for pelvic lists, and five-finger shoes for trail and off-trail walking and my feet and knees don't hurt anymore. I wear ONLY zero-drop shoes and I never wear shoes in my house. Now I stand (but not "still") in a pan filled with rocks on the floor in front of my standing workstation. Life = Revolutionized!

PAMELA ZAPOL THEDOS

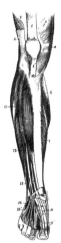

CHAPTER NINE

ADDING NATURAL SURFACES TO YOUR WALK

It's not just the little parts of you that need to be challenged—the very way you've been walking needs to be "strengthened" as well. The following are walking drills to assist your transition not only to better footwear, but to natural surfaces. If you're wearing minimal shoes for your health, then you must consider the spectrum of walking nutrients necessary for humans and not overdose on vitamin Flat and Level. Varying up your walking experience is key to ensuring you're not creating a repetitive environment for your newly awakened muscles. Therefore it is my suggestion that to keep feet functioning well, you expose them to other nutrients.

STONE-WALKING

Unlike your toes' muscles and joints, which can be stimulated by toe-lifting exercises, the joints of the foot "work" when deformed by what's underfoot.

In the natural world, your feet would be made supple through the organic relationship of lots of walking and lots of varied terrain—two elements that are missing from the modern world. If you really want to use more of your feet—more of your whole body, even—you have to walk on natural surfaces.

Sand, rocky paths, dirt paths, and root-filled forest floors are all nutritional input that mobilize the feet in unique ways. But while you need this input, your feet have significantly atrophied—which means you need to progress smartly.

To do so, you'll need texture. You can buy cobblestone mats, or find a playground with loose pebble fill, or even buy a bag of river rocks at your hardware store and put them either outside or on a mat inside. Before you walk, I suggest you stand on these surfaces. Instead of starting barefoot, take to new surfaces in your minimal shoes first, then socks, then barefoot. This way your joints will be buffered from the full impact of the joint deformation, which is another way of transitioning gradually. Listen to your feet and don't overdo it. The next stage would be walking on these same surfaces, which increases the loads to the feet quite a bit. While you create g-force acceleration of 1G (a load equal to your body weight) when standing, it's easy to create up to 1.75Gs while walking—a weight equal to 1.75 times your body weight—and 2–3Gs when running. This is why "barefoot training" should start with your shoes on.

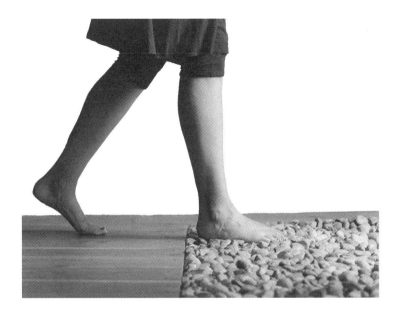

I like to keep a cobblestone mat in a hallway I walk down many times a day or at my standing desk area. This way I don't have to take any extra time out of my day to innervate all my intrinsic muscles.

Though it can feel like torture at first, if you expose your feet to these varied surfaces enough, you might even start to crave the sensation.

WALK ON THE PILLOW TRAIN

Just as your feet have been missing a wide range of stimulation (read: muscles' work and resulting adaptations) by walking on well-groomed ground, your ankles have been chronically overfed flat-and-level, and underfed all the other degrees of deformation necessary for varying slope, squatting, climbing trees, etc. Specific to walking, modern ankles are missing all the ways they would have been deformed had you been walking up and down hills, along sideways-sloping terrain, and over larger items like logs and rocks—which means when we do encounter the occasional hole or crack in our super flat world, we're totally unable to deal with it without injury.

Pillow-walking is a great exercise to gently and safely introduce the muscles of your feet and ankles to uneven and unstable terrain.

Make a short "train" of different pillows and cushions on your floor—throw pillows, couch cushions, a yoga bolster, and even folded-up towels will work for this. Walk back and forth across the pillows and feel your feet and ankles waking up. Bonus: If you have kids, they'll love this too—perfect for a rainy day when you're trapped inside.

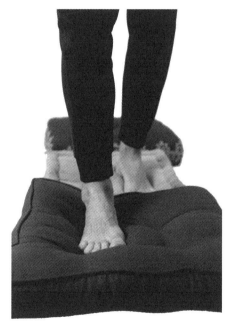

WALKING OVER VARIED TERRAIN

The best way to get a zillion joint angles in your feet, ankles, knees, and hips is to walk over natural, varied terrain. Think hilly forest trails littered with twigs, roots, and stones; a sloping meadow dotted with animal holes and thick clumps of plants; a rocky beach. Move your body through natural places and your feet will start experiencing the world the way our ancestors' feet did. You might not be able to take a long natural-terrain hike immediately, but you can start by leaving the main path for five or ten minutes at a time, and eventually you'll be able to go for hours.

Can't find long stretches of natural terrain? Don't feel limited by your urban jungle; when you're in the city, you can often find *more* varied alternatives to a flat and level sidewalk. If there's a grassy or dirt-patch verge between the sidewalk and the road, go ahead and walk on it. Is it flat, flat, flat for days? Take your hike to a skate park. Seriously! I know this stuff can sound like small potatoes, but slight movement variations—even the quick muscle responses to the most manicured of grassy surfaces—can be a big deal to an under-moved body.

" I had flat feet my whole life. All my ballet shoes from when I was a kid had solid grey soles. I was jealous of the other little kids who had "footprint-shaped" wear on the bottom of their ballet shoes. Then in my late thirties I transitioned to minimal footwear per your suggestions, diligently doing the exercises and going through different types of successively more minimal shoes up to the most minimal type I could find, every day. Now, in my forties, for the first time in my life I don't have flat feet anymore. When I pad back into the house barefoot with wet feet, I leave "footprint-shaped" footprints and I smile like a lunatic."

SARAH DE VRIES

" I have been a ballet teacher for over thirty years. Because of the demands of my job and the extreme repetitive use, I began experiencing pain in my feet, specifically my great toe joint. I have been doing barefoot restorative work for a year now and have found it extremely beneficial, restoring full articulation and relief. My wife and I walk our dog twice daily, go barefoot, and make a concerted eff ort to walk on a variety of surfaces."

STELIO CALAGIAS

WHOLE BODY BAREFOOT

VITAMIN TEXTURE?

In many cases, pediatric toe walking is idiopathic—meaning scientists and healthcare practitioners don't know why this particular gait pattern occurs. However, recent insights were made during a trial experiment that consisted of having toe-walking kids walk barefoot over different surfaces: gravel, carpet, and a laboratory floor. (Check out Fanchiang, H. D., M. D. Geil, J. Wu, T. Ajisafe, and Y. Chen, 2016, in the references, to read the whole fascinating study.) When walking over gravel, the heel height of the toe walkers decreased, leading the researchers to believe that exposing feet to texture could be a novel treatment for idiopathic toe walking.

On one hand I am glad for the potential of a non-invasive, inexpensive, and easily accessible therapy for toe-walking patients. On the other, I find myself asking, have researchers discovered a new therapy for toe walking, or have they discovered that toe walking is a sign of a missing "movement nutrient"?

In the 1700s, James Lind discovered that lemons or oranges could cure scurvy in sailors. But as you know, the big "takeaway science lesson" from that experiment wasn't that citrus fruits are a therapy for those with scurvy. The lesson was that foods containing vitamin C (later discovered by chemist Albert Szent-Györgyi in the 1930s) are essential for human function. Scurvy was simply the extreme manifestation of vitamin C deficiency that prompted the inquiry.

So, should we think of texture walking as a therapy for toe walkers, or does it make sense—considering the design of the foot, our understanding of how nerves and the balance systems of the body function, and evolutionary biology—that texture walking could be a requirement for optimal gait development?

You probably don't have scurvy, yet you know that you still require regular doses of vitamin C. Without it, you will begin to develop signs of deficiency. And while you might not toe walk, you might be showing signs of a texture deficiency in the form of more subtle (perhaps non-gait-related) symptoms. This most recent investigation of toe walkers strengthens the already biologically plausible argument that your body requires regular doses of vitamin Texture.

CHAPTER TEN

FIX YOUR FEET ALL DAY

I've been writing about foot turnout for years and noting that there's an alignment to the leg as a walking structure (foot to hip) that's best served by pointing the foot forward. Only, this process is not always as simple as turning your feet in, as not all turnouts are created the same way.

In general there are three ways of making a turnout, but also keep in mind that your turnout is likely a combination of the three. (Also, I'm numbering for clarity; the numbers have no clinical significance.)

Turnout One comes from the hips. In this case, your thigh-bones are turned outward and away from each other, as are the shin and foot. Looking at the legs from behind, the feet turn away from the midline, as do the knees. The upper leg and lower leg are "neutral" relative to each other. When the knees bend, the thigh moves in the direction of the outward-pointing foot. My brother, who fancies himself a cowboy, has this particular leg arrangement. When he walks his legs don't swing straight forward, but come out on a slight diagonal.

Turnout Two comes from the lower half of the knee. In this case, the shanks (lower legs) rotate away from the midline but the thighs still flex and extend in the sagittal plane (straight forward and back). This upper/lower leg relationship is a "medial moment" maker of the knee, which means when you bend your knee (in walking, going up and down stairs, and landing jumps), your thighbone moves along a different plane than your shin and foot. Not so fun for the medial structures (meniscus and anterior cruciate ligaments of the knee).

When you bend your knees in this position, the thigh bone moves in a plane that brings the knees together when they bend. Or, if you look at this arrangement from the back, you'll see that the knee pits look straight when the feet are pointing out. This is a classic "knock-kneed" orientation, although some feet are so turned out the knees are kept from touching.

Turnout Three looks practically identical to Turnout Two, but instead, the lower leg "turnout" is created by a turn *in the bone itself.* This is the most "permanent" turnout, but it is still helpful to understand bone robusticity—that is, how the shape of bone is affected by how you use it.

While we all have a basic bone shape that's consistent across the animal kingdom (if you can recognize a human femur then you're likely to be able to recognize the femur of a bird as well as a tiger), the nuance of bone is created by how a bone is used over a lifetime. In *Move Your DNA* I used professional baseball pitchers as my example (although the same phenomenon is found in volleyball and swimming athletes as well). In the case of professional pitchers, CT scans have shown that the throwing-arm bones of a pitcher are slightly twisted in the direction of their windup.

Imagine the windup necessary to throw a pitch. What a pitcher is doing is creating a series of "twists"—some large, at the hips and shoulder, some smaller, at the elbow and wrist—that he will unwind all at once, putting all that untwisting energy into the ball as it leaves the hand. Only, the ball isn't the only thing being thrown around. The cells in the pitcher's arm, too, are thrown around during the windup, and via a process called mechanotransduction, the bone takes a slightly new shape based on this mechanical input. So why am I putting pitchers and arm bones into this book about feet? Your cells are constantly being thrown about by how you move, and when it comes to gait (how you walk), you've taken a hundred million steps towards the bone shape you have now.

Torsion is defined as the twisting of an object along its own axis, where one end is moving relative to the opposite end; *rotation* is the turning of an entire unit about an axis.

While slight torsion is a natural phenomenon, populations with different movement behaviors, like those found in India and Japan, are known to have significantly less tibial torsion than those of European descent. This difference in bone shape is believed to be the result of loads to the bones created by squatting and floor sitting, which Europeans have largely missed out on. In fact, pediatric orthopedists and physios recommend children sit in different ways (swapping W-sitting for "criss-cross applesauce" or cross-legged sitting) because the loads in W-sitting can torque bones, potentially increasing both femur (thigh bone) and lower leg torsions. The takeaway? Loads (read: whole-body, whole-life movement) matter when it comes to the end-shape of your bones.

But let's say there is no end-shape, and what you've got right now is your shape, and you want to change it. Great. The point of this section is, while we need to un-duck our feet, this process is different for everyone and any progress is good progress, even if it's shifting the loads to your bones in teeny tiny steps.

On page 60 we direct you to straighten your feet during exercises, and this will become easier through doing all the exercises we've listed, but in the case of lower leg rotation and tibial torsion, there are some habit modifications and bodywork that can facilitate the process.

There are other things that we do that promote this lower leg turn-out and if you want to make progress, you have to consider how you're pushing your cells around all the time. Here are some of the behaviors I stopped doing when I realized they were impeding my own personal progress; you might realize you're doing slight variations of these once you start paying attention to how you move your feet and legs throughout the day.

- I uncrossed my ankles. It's totally natural to default to our comfort poses—crossing your arms in front, holding your wrists behind you, shifting your weight onto one leg, and slouching—because they're comfortable and save the body energy in the short term. One habit I'm super-diligent about catching (when I'm being super-diligent) is uncrossing my ankles. After years of working on my left shin I noticed, after an hour of foot and ankle work, that I was reading a book with my ankles crossed, putting my shin in the exact position I had just labored to get it out of. Now I uncross every time I catch myself.

- I stopped throwing my shins under the bus. Quick, go sit cross-legged on the floor. Use a few pillows if necessary. Now, look at your lower leg. Did you point your toes and roll onto the outside of the foot? Did you notice that you had to turn your lower leg out as well? When we take our unnaturally shaped bodies to a natural behavior like floor sitting, it's important to remember that the way we accomplish that natural movement is affected. So, in addition to bolstering tight hips, one might also think of bolstering the ankles as well, to not allow an exercise for the hips to take the lower leg. (And along the way you might realize that your leg as a whole isn't as mobile as you thought it was!)

- I stopped driving my feet wonky. It's not only shoes that have us on our toes; check out your feet next time you're driving your car and you're likely to find that you're spending quite a bit of time in plantarflexion. Make over your drive by making sure you're not pushing the pedals with a clenching foot or toes and instead create a smoother push.

Remember there's nothing actually wrong per se with gripping your toes on the gas, crossing the ankles, or sickling (the ballet term for pointing and rolling the foot to the outside); it's only that when you frequent those positions, they reinforce the old version of your body.

W-SITTING: YOU ARE HOW YOU MOVE

On the opposite page is a picture of my niece W-sitting. Anatomically speaking, a W-sit is created by a significant (some say excessive) internal rotation of the thigh bone coupled with a significant/excessive external rotation of the lower leg bones.

While she's clearly not pitching any baseballs in this image, she is pitching her cells in directions that can promote an end-distribution of mass that is a combination of Turnout Two and Turnout Three (discussed on page 114).

While there's a general consensus in the allopathic community regarding loads created via this position to be "bad," there is also a side to the debate that goes something like "all human positions are natural, so lay off the W-sitters."

Like the minimal footwear movement debate, I concur with both sides. In the end I would say that debating the issue

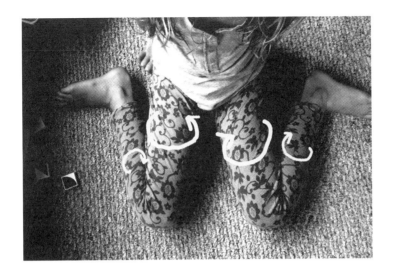

requires that we broaden the discussion to include all movements over a lifetime. Our unique culture has us shod and sitting at unprecedentedly high levels; the resulting "natural" preferences can be adaptations to the unnaturalness of our bodies. If one were W-sitting in the context of walking miles a day and doing all sorts of other leg motions, the twist-in-the-bone loads would be insignificant and the adaptation would be to a broader load profile. In the end, I'll just recommend that you take a look at the shape and functions of your body, see how they're working for you, and choose future movements based on your own "body of evidence."

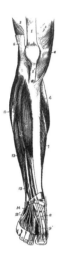

CONCLUSION

Believe it or not, I struggled for days over a hyphen. Whole-Body Barefoot or Whole Body Barefoot? I couldn't decide. When you have a compound adjective immediately preceding the thing being described, you hyphenate (according to my husband and my editor who know about such things). But, because the title wasn't ambiguous, they gave me permission to leave off the "-" as it didn't change the meaning of the words, and besides, they agreed it looked kind of funny.

But hyphen aside (sorry grammar zealots), I hope that, at this point, the title was clear—what you wear on your feet is a whole-body issue and not limited to the feet at all. Because you are not one single body, but a body fashioned out of trillions of smaller cellular bodies, the shoe you put on is never going on just your foot. You're putting that shoe onto a body of a trillion cells. And likewise, when you change your shoes, every cell in your body feels it.

I've taught thousands of people about their bodies and I always start with the feet. This is not because I have a foot fetish, but because, like you, I'm pressed for time. I'd love it if everyone carved time in their life to study how their body works, as well as time to implement what they know they need to do for optimal, whole-body function, but I'm a realist. We have busy lives and we have to prioritize many of life's essentials. Which is why I start with the foot. Most of you will be putting something onto your feet almost every day of your life. Shouldn't it be something that makes all trillion of you feel good?

THE MOVES

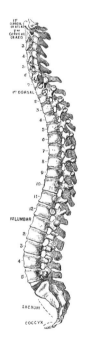

STANCE MOVES

ALIGN YOUR FEET

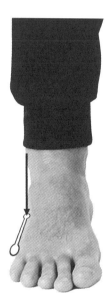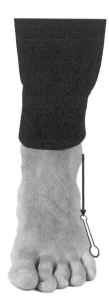

- To the best of your ability, align the outer edges of each foot using the points shown: the bony prominence just behind the little toe and the other a spot on the foot found by dropping an imaginary vertical line from the outer ankle bone to the floor.

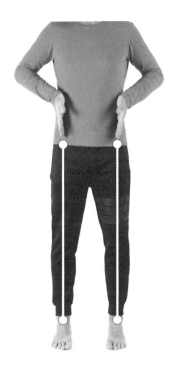

- Line up the center of the front of your ankles with the bony prominences at the front of your pelvis.

BACK YOUR HIPS UP

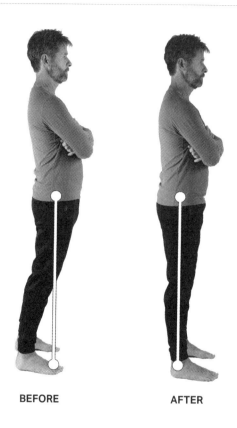

BEFORE   **AFTER**

- Move your hips back so that they're directly over the knees and ankles.

NEUTRAL FEMURS

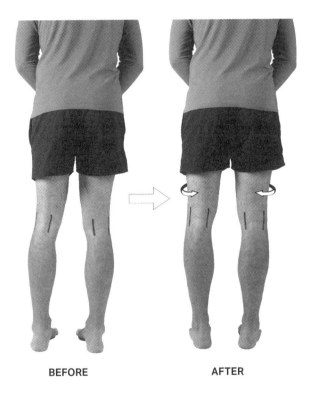

BEFORE **AFTER**

- Maintaining the above stance directions, rotate your femurs
  until your knee pits are pointing straight behind you.

INTRINSIC STRETCHES

PASSIVE TOE SPREADING

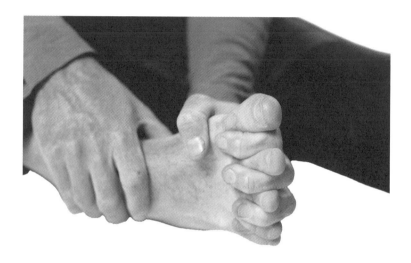

- Sit with one ankle crossed over the opposite knee.

- With your hands, gently spread your toes apart, stretching the toes away from each other.

- Hold for up to a minute at a time.

- Also try toe spacers and foot alignment socks.

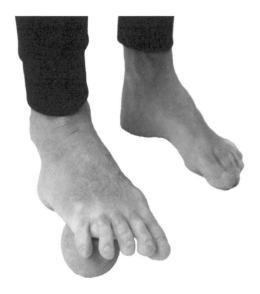

- Stand with a tennis or similarly sized squishy ball under the arch of one foot.

- Slowly load your weight (stay seated if necessary) onto the ball.

- Move your foot forward and back and side to side ("vacuuming" your foot) to gently articulate individual joints within the foot.

- Eventually try different ball sizes and firmness.

TOP OF THE FOOT STRETCH

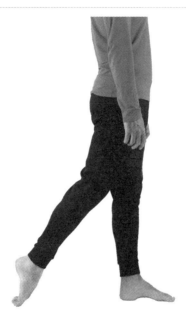

- Stand on your right foot and reach your left foot back behind you, tucking the toes of your left foot under and placing them on the floor.

- If you find yourself leaning forward, shorten the distance you've reached the leg back.

- Bring your pelvis over your standing ankle and upper body over the hips.

- Work up to holding this stretch for a minute, but stop for cramping.

EXTRINSIC STRETCHES

CALF STRETCH – GASTROCNEMIUS

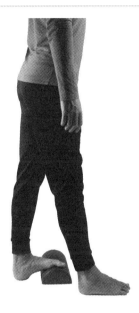

- Place the ball of your left foot on the apex of a half-foam roller or rolled-up folded towel, drop the heel all the way to the ground, and straighten that knee.

- Step forward with your right foot.

- If you can't bring your foot all the way forward, take a smaller step.

- Keep your weight stacked vertically over the heel of which ever foot is farther back.

- Hold for a minute, then switch legs; do this three times each leg.

CALF STRETCH – SOLEUS

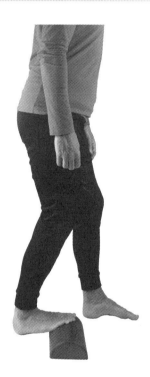

- After getting into Calf Stretch – Gastrocnemius position, bend the knees while keeping your heels down.

- Hold for up to a minute, then switch legs; repeat this as often as you do the Calf Stretch – Gastrocnemius.

DOUBLE CALF STRETCH

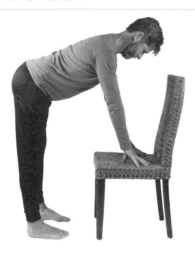

- Stand in front of a chair, facing the seat. With your feet pelvis-width apart, knees straight, and feet pointing forward, tip the pelvis forward until your palms rest on the chair.

- If you can't reach the chair without really bending the knees or rounding the back, make your seat height higher or move to a counter or desktop.

- Once your arms are down, see if you can allow your spine to drop down toward the floor, and your tailbone to lift toward the ceiling.

- Don't force your ribs to the floor or arch your back—just consciously relax the spine to the ground as much as you can.

- Hold for up to a minute and repeat often throughout the day.

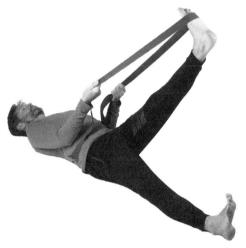

- Lie on your back and loop a strap (or a belt) across the toe-box of your right foot.

- Straighten your right leg above you and extend your left leg until your left hamstring is touching the floor.

- If you have to bring your right leg lower for the left hamstring to touch, do so, keeping both legs straight.

- Allow your arms to hold the weight of your right leg—relax it completely and then pull your foot toward you with the strap, not with the muscles down the front of the shin.

- Keeping your ankle in place, pull your right leg higher in small increments, without allowing the left hamstring to come up off the floor.

CATSUIT STRETCH

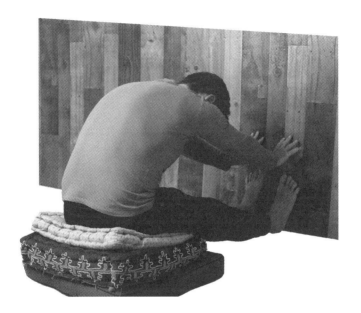

- Sit on the floor with your feet pressed flat against a wall and your legs straight.

- Fold your body forward, tipping your pelvis, ribs, and chest towards your legs.

- Completely relax your neck, letting your head hang.

CALF STACK

- **Stack one**: Sitting on the floor or a cushion, bring one bent leg in front of your body, placing a ball beneath the outside of your shin. Stack a second ball on top and hold in place with your hand.

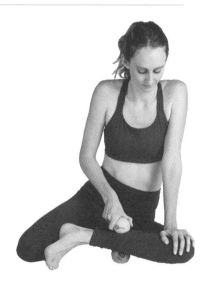

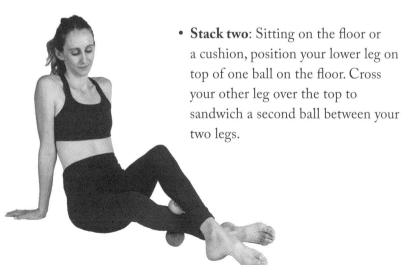

- **Stack two**: Sitting on the floor or a cushion, position your lower leg on top of one ball on the floor. Cross your other leg over the top to sandwich a second ball between your two legs.

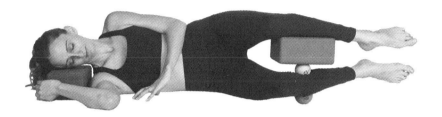

- **Stack three**: Lie on your side with a pillow beneath your head, hips and knees bent to 90°. Stack one ball on the floor under your first leg, then stack a second ball on top, pinning it with a block and your other leg on top.

- In all stacks, point, flex, and circle your ankles and feet, then re-stack the balls higher or lower along your lower leg and repeat.

INTRINSIC STRENGTHENERS

TOE ABDUCTION

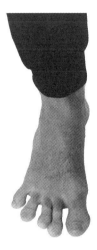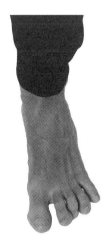

- Stand with your feet pelvis-width apart and pointing straight ahead, and your weight back in your heels.

- Spread your toes apart as far as you can, keeping all the toes flat on the ground.

- Repeat throughout the day (read: make sure your shoes aren't too tight to do this motion!).

TOE LIFTS

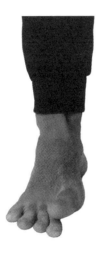 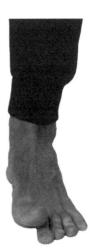

- Lift just your big toes while in the same stance as the last exercise.

- Work to lift each big toe straight upward, rather than sideways across the foot.

- Lift first the big toes and then the second toe of each foot, making sure to keep the balls of your feet on the floor. Then lift the third, fourth, and fifth toes.

- Once all the toes are lifted, put them back down one by one.

EXTRINSIC STRENGTHENERS

SINGLE-LEG BALANCE

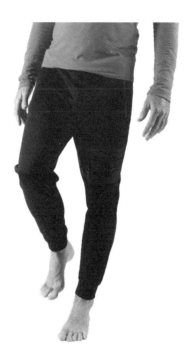

- Stand barefoot on the left leg with the knee straight and bend the right knee to lift the right foot slightly off the floor.

- Keep your ankle still, your arms down by your sides, and your foot pointing straight ahead (with knee pits facing back, once you're more advanced).

- Hold for up to a minute on each side, three times each.

SINGLE-LEG TOWEL BALANCE

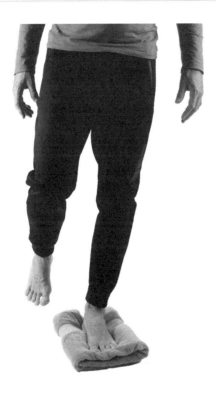

- Repeat the single-leg balance while standing on a folded towel.

- Balance for up to one minute before switching legs.

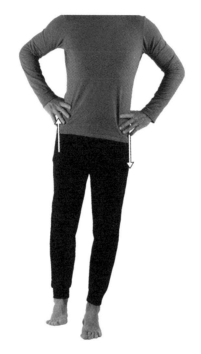

- Standing in neutral—feet straight, ankles pelvis-width apart, weight on the rear of the foot—place your right hand on your right hip and pull the right side of the pelvis down toward the floor, bringing the left side up.

- Neither knee bends during this exercise.

- Hold for up to a minute on each side.

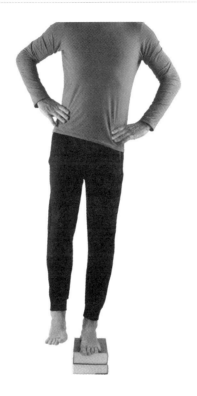

- Perform the List while standing on a phone book or yoga block with the other leg floating above the ground.

- Work up to doing this for six minutes, alternating sides every minute.

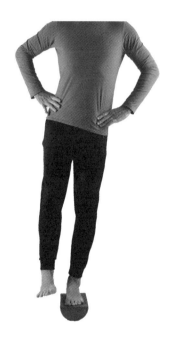

- This is the same as the Next-Level List, but it's performed on an inverted half-foam roller.

- Try to attain a neutral knee pit while listing.

- Work up to doing this for six minutes, alternating sides every minute.

- Eventually, the listing action should occur naturally while you're walking.

CALF ELEVATORS

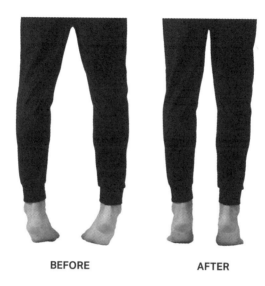

BEFORE   **AFTER**

- Stand with your feet forward, ankles pelvis-width apart.

- Slowly lift your heels away from the ground without overly moving your pelvis forward.

- Keep your ankles straight (don't let them drop outward, as in top left photo) and continuously press the ball of the foot into the floor.

- Lift and lower your heels, working up to twenty times.

- Eventually work up to doing this exercise one foot at a time.

TERRAIN TRAINING

STONE-WALKING

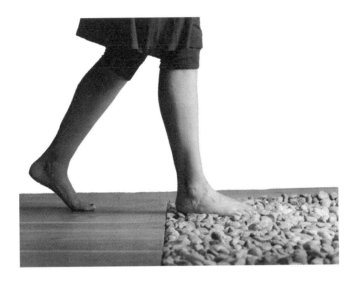

- Begin by standing in minimal footwear (then socks, then barefoot as you become used to the sensation) on stones or cobblestone mat.

- Progress slowly to walking barefoot on these surfaces.

WHOLE BODY BAREFOOT

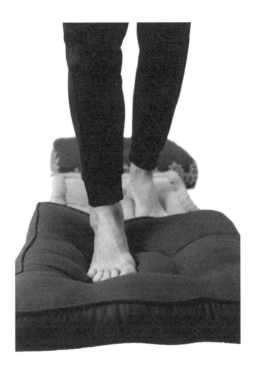

- Make a short "train" of different pillows and cushions on your floor.

- Walk back and forth across the pillows.

APPENDICES

APPENDIX ONE: HOW TO SHOP FOR MINIMAL SHOES

The first step to shopping for minimal shoes is finding them! With companies and styles coming and going all the time, I maintain an updated list of minimal/transitioning-to-minimal shoe companies on my website, broken down into categories like season, children, and special occasion (yes, you can wear minimal shoes to a wedding!).

Mimimal shoe list: nutritiousmovement.com/shoes-the-list

There are also plenty of shoe styles that qualify as minimal, even though they weren't made to be minimal, so you don't need to limit your choices to minimal footwear brands. I often find shoes that are flat and flexible poking around regular shoe stores, so it's best to shop for shoes by minimal footwear characteristics: heel height, toe-box width, elevated toe-box, upper, and sole. On the opposite page is a useful chart from my book *Simple Steps to Foot Pain Relief* that shows the range of each shoe element.

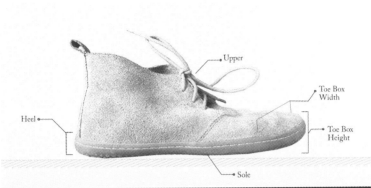

Upper

Toe Box
Width

Heel

Toe Box
Height

Sole

ELEMENT	BEST	NOT TOO BAD	RESTRICTS BODY MOVEMENT	
HEEL	Flat	Minimal positive, below ¼"	Positive, 1-2"	Positive, more than 2"
TOE-BOX WIDTH	Toes move freely	Toes have some space	Toes can't move	Toes are squished
TOE-BOX HEIGHT	Flat	Slight lift before your foot is in	Elevated while standing	Elevated and stiff
UPPER	Well attached	Sandal with heel strap	Slide	Flip-flop
SOLE	Thin and flexible	Flexible, even if not so thin	Rigid, even if not so thick	Thick and rigid

APPENDICES

When transitioning towards less external foot/leg support, you can choose which footwear elements you'd like to start with. We need to choose the right shoe for our body right now—the same minimal shoe or minimal shoe elements won't be right for every body and lifestyle. Maybe you stand all day for work, in which case getting rid of a heel would be impactful, but getting rid of a thicker sole would not feel great. In this case, you'd look for a shoe that was flat but had some cushion in the sole.

Out of all the "minimal" characteristics a shoe can have, I have found it easiest to find non-heeled shoes. While minimal shoes tend to have more toe-box space than conventional shoes, many minimal styles still have a narrow toe-boxes compared to the width your toes will eventually occupy.

Take your new understanding of footwear attributes into a shoe store, and you might find the right shoe for you!

SHOE SIZING

As in regular footwear, minimal shoe sizing isn't standard. Try on many styles of shoes to get a feel for what you need exactly. And know that as you do your corrective exercises and habit modifications, the size and shape of your foot will change. What works for you this week might not work in a year.

One great tip for selecting an appropriate toe-box width is to trace your bare foot—with your toes spread as much as possible—on paper and then place a potential shoe on top of the drawing to see how they compare. This is one way to see the potential restrictions your shoe might be placing on your toe spreading.

If you're going to be walking or running in your shoes, try them on after a walk or a run, or at the end of the day when your feet are the largest. If a shoe doesn't feel good in the store, you likely need a different style or size. Finding a comfortable shoe up front will save you time, money, and foot aches in the long run (or walk).

APPENDIX TWO: RESOURCES TO KEEP YOUR FEET AND WHOLE BODY MOVING MORE

Half-foam roller (6"x3"x12")
nutritiousmovement.com/product/half-dome

Correct Toes
nwfootankle.com/correct-toes

Alignment Socks
my-happyfeet.com

Toe Spacers
earthrunners.com/products/toe-spacers

Yoga Tune Up® Balls
yogatuneup.com

Simple Steps To Foot Pain Relief: The New Science of Healthy Feet by Katy Bowman (BenBella Books)
   This is a book all about how and why to choose better footwear.

The Roll Model: A Step-by-Step Guide to Erase Pain, Improve Mobility, and Live Better in Your Body by Jill Miller (Victory Belt Publishing)

OTHER WAYS TO LEARN FROM ME

Social Media
You can find years of visual insights into a movement-rich life here: instagram.com/nutritiousmovement

My Podcast:
You can listen to the award-winning *Move Your DNA* (another way to learn on the move) on iTunes, Stitcher, or on my website nutritiousmovement.com, where you can also find transcripts of the show.

Exercise Classes/Videos:
Visit nutritiousmovement.com to find out more about the live and recorded classes I teach as well as my exercise DVDs, downloadable classes, and movement courses or to find a movement teacher in your area trained in these moves.

REFERENCES AND
FURTHER READING

Arnadottir, S., and V. Mercer. 2000. Effects of footwear on measurements of balance and gait in women between the ages of 65 and 93 years. *Physical Therapy* 80 (1): 17-27.

Barnett, C. 1962. The normal orientation of the human hallux and the effect of footwear. *Journal of Anatomy* 96 (Part 4): 489-94.1.

Barnicot, N.A. 1955. The position of the hallux in West Africans. *Journal of Anatomy* 89 (Part 3): 355–61.

Bendix, T., S. Sorensen, and K. Klausen. 1984. Lumbar curve, trunk muscles, and line of gravity with different heel heights. *Spine* 9 (2): 223-27.

Bergmann, G., H. Kniggendorf, F. Graichen, and A. Rohlmann. 1995. Influence of shoes and heel strike on the loading of the hip joint. *Journal of Biomechanics* 28 (7): 817-27.

Birn-Jeffery, A.V., and T.E. Higham. 2014. The scaling of uphill and downhill locomotion in legged animals. *Integrative and Comparative Biology*. [Epub ahead of print]

Carl, T., S. Barrett. 2008. Computerized analysis of plantar pressure variation in flip-flops, athletic shoes, and bare feet. *Journal of the American Podiatric Medical Association* 98 (5): 374-78.

Carpenter, K.J. 2012. The discovery of vitamin C. *Annals of Nutrition and Metabolism* 61(3): 259-64.

Chevalier, Gaétan, S. T. Sinatra, J. L. Oschman, K. Sokal, and P. Sokal. 2012. Earthing: health implications of reconnecting the human body to the Earth's surface electrons. *Journal of Environmental and Public Health,* Article ID 291541: 1-8.

Cho, N.H., S. Kim, D.J. Kwon, and H.A. Kim. 2009. The prevalence of hallux valgus and its association with foot pain and function in a rural Korean community. *Journal of Bone and Joint Surgery*—British Volume 91 (4): 494-98.

Crockett, H., B. Gross, K. Wilk, M. Schwartz, J. Reed, J. O'Mara & J. Andrews. 2000. Osseous adaptation and range of motion at the gleno-humeral joint in professional baseball. *The American Journal of Sports Medicine* 30 (1): 20-26.

Csapo, R., C. Maganaris, O. Seynnes, and M. Narici. 2010. On muscle, tendon and high heels. *Journal of Experimental Biology* 213: 2582-88.

Daoût, K., T. Pataky, D. De Clercq, and P. Aerts. 2009. The effects of habitual footwear use: foot shape and function in native barefoot walkers. *Footwear Science* 1 (2): 81-94.

Dawson, J., M. Thorogood, S. Marks, E. Juszczak, C. Dodd, G. Lavis, and R. Fitzpatrick. 2002. The prevalence of foot problems in older women: a cause for concern. *Journal of Public Health* 24 (2): 77-84.

de Lateur, B., R. Giaconi, K. Questad, M. Ko, and J. Lehmann. 1991. Footwear and posture: compensatory strategies for heel height. *American Journal of Physical Medicine Rehabilitation* 70 (5): 246-54.

De Wit, B., D. De Clercq, and P. Aerts. 2000. Biomechanical analysis of the stance phase during barefoot and shod running. *Journal of Biomechanics* 33 (3): 269-78.

Eisenhardt, J., D. Cook, I. Pregler, and H. Foehl. 1996. Changes in temporal gait characteristics and pressure distribution for bare feet versus various heel heights. *Gait and Posture* 4 (4): 280-86.

Esenyel, M., K. Walsh, J. Walden, A. Gitter. 2003. Kinetics of high-heeled gait. *Journal of the American Podiatric Medical Association* 93 (1): 27-32.

Fanchiang, H. D., M. D. Geil, J. Wu, T. Ajisafe, and Y. Chen. 2016. "The Effects of Walking Surface on the Gait Pattern of Children With Idiopathic Toe Walking." *Journal of Child Neurology* 31(7): 858–63.

Frey, C., F. Thompson, J. Smith, M. Sanders, and H. Horstman. 1993. American Orthopedic Foot and Ankle Society women's shoe survey. *Foot and Ankle* 14 (2): 78-81.

Fulkerson, J., E. Arendt, L. Griffin, J. Garrick. 2002. Anterior knee pain in females. *Clinical Orthopedics & Related Research* 372 (March): 69-73.

Gabell, A., M. Simons, U. Nayak. 1985. Falls in the healthy elderly: predisposing causes. *Ergonomics* 28 (7): 965-75.

Gefen, A., M. Megido-Ravid, Y. Itzchak, and M. Arcan. 2001. Analysis of muscular fatigue and foot stability during high-heeled gait. *Gait and Posture* 15 (1): 56-63.

Giuliani, Jeffrey; B. Masini, C. Alitz, B. D. Owens. 2011. Bare-foot-simulating footwear associated with metatarsal stress injury in two runners. *Healio Orthopedics* 34 (7): e320-e323).

Gottschalk F., J. Sallis, P. Beighton, and L. Solomon. 1980. A comparison of the prevalence of hallux valgus in three South African populations. *South African Medical Journal* 57 (10): 355-57.

Hill, C., T. Gill, H. Menz, and A. Taylor. 2008. Prevalence and correlates of foot pain in a population-based study: the North West Adelaide health study. *Journal of Foot and Ankle Research*, July 28, 2008.

Jenkins, D. W. and D. J. Cauthon. 2011. Barefoot running claims and controversies. *Journal of the American Podiatric Medical Association* 101 (3): 231-246.

Kerrigan, D., J. Johansson, M. Bryant, J. Boxer, U. Croce, and P. Riley. 2005. Moderate-heeled shoes and knee joint torques relevant to the development and progression of knee osteoarthritis. *Physical Medicine and Rehabilitation* 86 (5): 871-75.

Kerrigan, D., J. Lelas, and M. Karvosky. 2001. Women's shoes and knee osteoarthritis. *The Lancet* 357 (9262): 1097-98.

Kerrigan, D., M. Todd, and P. Riley. 1998. Knee osteoarthritis and high-heeled shoes. *The Lancet* 351 (9113): 1399-1401.

Kirby, K. A. 2001. Subtalar joint axis location and rotational equilibrium theory of foot function. *Journal of the American Podiatric Medical Association* 91 (9): 465-487.

Lee, C., E. Jeong, and A. Freivalds. 2001. Biomechanical effects of wearing high-heeled shoes. *International Journal of Industrial Ergonomics* 28 (6): 321-26.

Lieberman, Daniel E., M. Venkadesan, W.A. Werbel, A. I. Daoud, S. D'Andrea, I.S. Davis, R. Ojiambo Mang'Eni & Y. Pitsiladis. 2010. Foot strike patterns and collision forces in habitually barefoot versus shod runners. *Nature* 463: 531-535.

Maclennan, R. 1966. Prevalence of hallux valgus in a neolithic New Guinea population. *The Lancet* 287 (7452): 1398-1400.

Martin, R. Bruce, Burr, David B., & Sharkey, Neil A. 1998. *Skeletal Tissue Mechanics.* New York: Springer-Verlag.

McBride I., U. Wyss, T. Cooke, L. Murphy, J. Phillips, and S. Olney. 1991. First metatarsophalangeal joint reaction forces during high-heel gait. *Foot and Ankle* 11 (5): 282-88.

Menz, H.B., and M.E. Morris. 2005. Footwear characteristics and foot problems in older people. *Gerontology* 51 (5): 346-51.

Menz, H.B., A. Tiedemann, M.M. Kwan, K. Plumb, and S.R. Lord. 2007. Foot pain in community-dwelling older people: an evaluation of the Manchester Foot Pain and Disability Index. *Rheumatology* (Oxford) 46 (2): 375.

Morgan, Christopher. 2008. Reconstructing prehistoric hunter-gatherer foraging radii: a case study from California's southern Sierra Nevada. *Journal of Archaeological Science* 35 (2): 247-258.

Mullaji A.B., A.K. Sharma, S.V. Marawar, A. F. Kohli. 2008. Tibial torsion in non-arthritic Indian adults: A computer tomography study of 100 limbs. *Indian Journal of Orthopaedics* 42 (3): 309-13.

Nigg, B. 2001. The role of impact forces and foot pronation: a new paradigm. *Clinical Journal of Sports Medicine* 11 (1): 2-9.

Nix, S., M. Smith, and B. Vicenzino. 2010. Prevalence of hallux valgus in the general population: a systematic review and meta-analysis. *Journal of Foot and Ankle Research* 3 (September 27): 21.

Nurse, M.A., et al. 2005. Changing the texture of footwear can alter gait patterns. *Journal of Electromyography and Kinesiology* 15 (5): 496-506.

Raichlen, D.A., B.M. Wood, A.D. Gordon, A.Z. Mabulla, F.W. Marlowe and H. Pontzer. 2014. Evidence of Levy walk foraging patterns in human hunter-gatherers. *Proceedings of the National Academy of Sciences* 111(2): 728-33.

Rao, U., and B. Joseph. 1992. The influence of footwear on the prevalence of flat foot. A survey of 2300 children. *The Journal of Bone and Joint Surgery* 74 (4): 525-27.

Ridge, Sarah T.; Johnson, A. Wayne; Mitchell, Ulrike H.; Hunter, Iain; Robinson, Eric; Rich, Brent S. E.; Brown, Stephen Douglas. 2013. Foot bone marrow edema after 10-week transition to minimalist running shoes. *Medicine & Science in Sports & Exercise* 45 (7): 1363-8.

Rixe, Jeffrey A., R.A. Gallo, M.L. Silvis. 2012. The barefoot debate: can minimalist shoes reduce running-related injuries? *Current Sports Medicine Report* 11 (3): 160-65.

Robbins, S., and A. Hanna. 1987. Running-related injury prevention through barefoot adaptations. *Medicine and Science in Sports and Exercise* 19 (2): 148-56.

Robbins, S., G. Gouw, and A. Hanna. 1989. Running-related injury prevention through innate impact-moderating behavior. *Medicine and Science in Sports and Exercise* 21 (2): 130-39.

Rome, K., D. Hancock, and D. Poratt. 2008. Barefoot running and walking: the pros and cons based on current evidence. *The New Zealand Medical Journal* 121 (1272).

Rossi, William A. 1999. Why shoes make 'normal' gait impossible. *Podiatry Management* (March): 50-61.

Rossi, W. 2001. Footwear: the primary cause of foot disorders. A continuation of the scientific review of the failings of modern shoes. *Podiatry Management* (February): 129-38.

Shaw, C.N. and Stock, J.T. 2009. Habitual throwing and swimming correspond with upper limb diaphyseal strength and shape in modern human athletes. *American Journal of Physical Anthropology* 140 (1): 160-172.

Sherrington, C., and H. Menz. 2002. An evaluation of footwear worn at the time of fall-related hip fracture. *Age and Aging* 32 (3): 310-14.

Shroyer, J., and W. Weimar. 2010. Comparative analysis of human gait while wearing thong-style flip-flops versus sneakers. *Journal of the American Podiatric Medical Association* 100 (4): 251-57.

Shull, P.B., R. Shultz, A. Slider, J.L. Dragoo, T.F. Besier and S. L. Delp. 2013. Toe-in gait reduces the first peak knee adduction moment in patients with medial compartment knee osteoarthritis. *Journal of Biomechanics*, 46 (1), 122-128.

Sládek, V., M. Berner, R. Sailer. 2006. Mobility in Central European Late Eneolithic and Early Bronze Age: Tibial Cross-sectional Geometry. *Journal of Archaeological Science* 33 (4): 470–482.

Venkataraman, V.V., T.S. Kraft, J.M. Desilva and N.J. Dominy. 2013. Phenotypic plasticity of climbing-related traits in the ankle joint of great apes and rainforest hunter-gatherers. *Human Biology*, 85(1-3): 309-28.

Venkataraman, V.V., T.S. Kraft and N.J. Dominy. 2013. Tree climbing and human evolution. *Proceedings of the National Academy of Sciences of the United States of America* 110 (4): 1237-42.

Villamin, C.A.C., and J.F.C. Syquia. 2012. Tibial torsion among Filipinos: a cavaderic study. *Malaysian Orthopedic Journal* 6 (3): 27-30.

von Tscharner, V., B. Goepfert, and B. Nigg. 2003. Changes in EMG signals for the muscle tibialis anterior while running barefoot or with shoes resolved by non-linearly scaled wavelets. *Journal of Biomechanics* 36 (8): 1169-76.

Vormittag, K., R. Calonje, and W.W. Briner. 2009. Foot and ankle injuries in the barefoot sport. *Current Sports Medicine Reports* 8 (5): 262-66.

Weist, Roger, E. Eils, D. Rosenbaum. 2004. The influence of muscle fatigue on electromyogram and plantar pressure patterns as an explanation for the incidence of metatarsal stress fractures. *American Journal of Sports Medicine* 32 (8): 1893-1898.

Willems, T., E. Witvrouw, A. De Cock, and D. De Clercq. 2007. Gait-related risk factors for exercise-related lower-leg pain during shod running. *Medicine and Science in Sports and Exercise* 39 (2): 330-39.

Zipfel, B. and L.R. Berger. 2007. Shod versus unshod: the emergence of forefoot pathology in modern humans. *The Foot* 17 (4): 205-13.

INDEX

M

McDougall, Christopher, 2

mechanotransduction, 25, 115

metatarsal, 34, 104

Miller, Jill, 88-90, 154

Move Your DNA, 25, 30, 115, 155

N

neuromas, 63

neutral femurs/knee pits (stance habit), 46, 52, **64-65**, 70, 99-101, 127, 144

next-level list, **100**, 143

next-next level list, **101**, 144

O

orthotic, 27, 37, 48, 52, 71, 94, 104

osteoarthritis, 62, 95

P

passive toe spreading, **67-69**, 92, 128

pelvic list, **99-100**, 104, 142

pelvic thrust, 62-63, 85

plantar fasciitis, 9, 48, 80

pronation, 16, 37-39, 48, 52

toe walking, 11-112

top of the foot stretch, 34, **72-74**, 94, 130

torsion, 115-116

turnout, 113-114, 118

U

un-duck your feet (*see* turnout)

upper (in footwear), **5**, 16, 29, 34, 150

V

vitamin Texture, 111-112

W

W-sitting, 118-119

walk on the pillow train, **107-108**, 147

walking over varied terrain, 18, 29, 43, 97, 102, 103, 106-108, **109**, 146-147

ABOUT THE AUTHOR

Bestselling author, speaker, and a leader of the Movement movement, biomechanist Katy Bowman is changing the way we move and think about our need for movement. Her ten books, including the groundbreaking *Move Your DNA*, have been translated into more than sixteen languages worldwide.

Bowman teaches movement globally and speaks about sedentarism and movement ecology to academic and scientific audiences such as the Ancestral Health Summit and the Institute for Human and Machine Cognition. Her work is regularly featured in diverse media such as the Today Show, CBC Radio One, the *Seattle Times,* the Joe Rogan Experience, and *Good Housekeeping*. One of Maria Shriver's "Architects of Change" and an America Walks "Woman of the Walking Movement," Bowman consults on educational and living space design to encourage movement-rich habitats. She has worked with companies like Patagonia, Nike, and Google as well as a wide range of non-profits and other communities to create greater access to her "move more, move more body parts, move more for what you need" message. Her movement education company, Nutritious Movement, is based in Washington State, where she lives with her family.

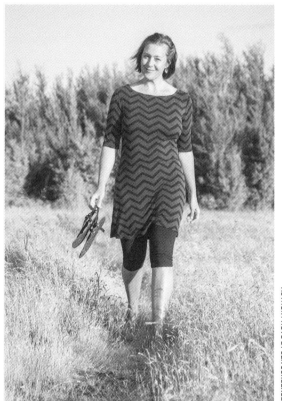

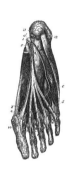